Helical (Spiral) Computed Tomography

A Practical Approach
To Clinical Protocols

Helical (Spiral) Computed Tomography
A Practical Approach To Clinical Protocols

Editor

Paul M. Silverman, M.D.

Professor of Radiology and Medical Oncology
Division of Abdominal Imaging
Director of Computed Tomography
Georgetown University Medical Center
Washington, D.C.

Contributors

James A. Brink

Philip Costello

Elliott K. Fishman

Jay P. Heiken

Anthony A. Mancuso

David P. Naidich

Geoffrey D. Rubin

Ilona M. Schmalfuss

Marilyn J. Siegel

Paul M. Silverman

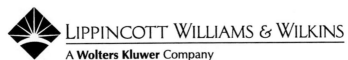

LIPPINCOTT WILLIAMS & WILKINS

A **Wolters Kluwer** Company

Philadelphia • Baltimore • New York • London
Buenos Aires • Hong Kong • Sydney • Tokyo

Acquisitions Editor: James D. Ryan
Developmental Editor: Michelle M. LaPlante
Manufacturing Manager: Dennis Teston
Production Manager: Jodi Borgenicht
Production Editor: Jeff Somers
Cover Designer: Keithley Associates
Indexer: Lisa Mullenneaux
Compositor: Maryland Composition
Printer: Quebecor Kingsport

Printed in the United States of America

9 8 7 6 5 4 3 2

Library of Congress Cataloging-in-Publication Data

Helical (spiral) computed tomography : a practical approach to
 clinical protocols / editor, Paul M. Silverman ; contributors, James
 A. Brink ... [et al.].
     p.   cm.
   Includes bibliographical references and index.
   ISBN 0-7817-1478-8 (alk. paper)
   1. Spiral computed tomography.   I. Silverman, Paul M.   II. Brink,
James A.
   [DNLM: 1. Tomography, X-Ray Computed—methods.   WN 206 H4749
1998]
RC78.7.T6H445   1998
616.07′572—dc21
DNLM/DLC
for Library of Congress   97-31575
                                                                CIP

Care has been taken to confirm the accuracy of the information presented and to describe generally accepted practices. However, the authors, editor, and publisher are not responsible for errors or omissions or for any consequences from application of the information in this book and make no warranty, express or implied, with respect to the contents of the publication.

The authors, editor, and publisher have exerted every effort to ensure that drug selection and dosage set forth in this text are in accordance with current recommendations and practice at the time of publication. However, in view of ongoing research, changes in government regulations, and the constant flow of information relating to drug therapy and drug reactions, the reader is urged to check the package insert for each drug for any change in indications and dosage and for added warnings and precautions. This is particularly important when the recommended agent is a new or infrequently employed drug.

Some drugs and medical devices presented in this publication have Food and Drug Administration (FDA) clearance for limited use in restricted research settings. It is the responsibility of the health care provider to ascertain the FDA status of each drug or device planned for use in their clinical practice.

To my wonderful wife Amy and my children, Zachary and
Rebecca, who bring true joy into my life.

Contents

Contributing Authors

James A. Brink, M.D. *Associate Professor of Radiology, Department of Radiology, Yale University School of Medicine, 333 Cedar Street, New Haven, Connecticut 06510*

Philip Costello, M.D., F.A.C.R. *Professor of Radiology, Director of Radiology, The Queen Elizabeth Hospital, Adelaide, South Australia 5011*

Elliott K. Fishman, M.D. *Department of Radiology, Johns Hopkins Hospital, 600 North Wolfe Street, Baltimore, Maryland 21287*

Jay P. Heiken, M.D. *Professor of Radiology, Mallinckrodt Institute of Radiology, Washington University School of Medicine, 510 South Kingshighway Boulevard, St. Louis, Missouri 63110*

Anthony A. Mancuso, M.D. *Professor of Radiology, Department of Radiology, University of Florida, College of Medicine, P.O. Box 100374, JHMHC, Gainesville, Florida 32610*

David P. Naidich, M.D. *Professor of Radiology, Director, Computed Tomography, Department of Radiology, Bellevue Hospital, 462 1st Avenue, New York, New York 10016*

Geoffrey D. Rubin, M.D. *Assistant Professor of Radiology, Department of Radiology, Stanford University School of Medicine, 300 Pasteur Drive, Room S072B, Stanford, California 94305*

Ilona M. Schmalfuss, M.D. *Department of Radiology, University of Florida, College of Medicine, 1600 SW Archer Road, Gainesville, Florida 32610*

Marilyn J. Siegel, M.D. *Professor of Radiology and Pediatrics, Department of Radiology, Mallinckrodt Institute of Radiology, Washington University School of Medicine, 510 South Kingshighway Boulevard, St. Louis, Missouri 63110*

Paul M. Silverman, M.D. *Professor of Radiology and Medical Oncology, Division of Abdominal Imaging, Director of Computed Tomography, Georgetown University Medical Center, 3800 Reservoir Road, N.W., Washington, D.C. 20007*

Preface

Since its introduction, helical (spiral) CT has had a dramatic impact upon the approach to CT scanning. The most obvious and direct impact has been in the increased speed of scanning. Technological advances which make this possible include slip-ring technology, improved detectors and tubes, and advanced computer hardware and software. This technology presents new challenges for physicians who must have a fundamental understanding of its differences from conventional CT in order to maximize its clinical impact. For example, new terms such as pitch require an appreciation of how this parameter can be varied to optimize various examinations. Rapid scanning effectively translates into markedly improved enhancement of parenchymal structures, detection of lesions, and the potential for more accurate staging of patients with malignancies. Helical (spiral) CT allows, for the first time, true three-dimensional (3-D) imaging, particularly of vascular structures, which enhances the planning of surgical procedures. Not only can vessels be evaluated for stenoses but vascular encasement by tumor can be readily displayed. The dramatic decrease in the price of high-level computer hardware and software has made developments in the area of virtual reality possible. Virtual endoscopy and colonoscopy have become a reality, although much work needs to be done to be able to establish specific protocols for clinical care. In addition, new hardware and software packages with computer-automated scanning allow for monitoring in almost real-time enhancement following intravenous contrast administration of target organs and vessels to optimize imaging without the use of a test bolus of contrast. This approach compensates for individual variations in the cardiac output, providing more consistent examinations from patient-to-patient and, in the case of liver examinations, allowing the use of less contrast material.

These advances have had a dramatic impact upon the way radiologists perform CT scanning. It is clear that helical (spiral) scanning will be the dominant technology for the future. With these advances comes the responsibility to use this equipment to its utmost. In converting from conventional to helical CT scanning, scanning protocols need revision, incorporating a full understanding of contrast dynamics, scan parameters, length of helical exposure, and the inter-relationships of collimation and pitch for generating high quality, three-dimensional (3-D) image displays. The goal of this book is to provide radiologists and their technologists with not only effective and practical protocols, but an appreciation of the rational approach used to generate these protocols.

Helical (Spiral) Computed Tomography: A Practical Approach to Clinical Protocols consists of a general introduction and six chapters. The following six areas are covered: head and neck, chest, abdomen and pelvis, musculoskeletal and bone, pediatrics, and three-dimensional (3-D) imaging. Each chapter has its own specific introduction which discusses the principles behind the recommended protocols. This is followed by a list of pertinent references from the literature. Following this is a comprehensive list of protocols for specific clinical indications. These are described in a detailed but easily readable outline form which includes the following:

SCANNING PROTOCOLS

    I. INDICATION: Anatomic region (clinical indication)
    II. SCANNER SETTINGS: kVp, mAs
    III. ORAL CONTRAST: Barium, Gastrograffin, negative contrast agent
    IV. PHASE OF RESPIRATION: Inspiration, expiration, selective maneuvers
    V. SLICE THICKNESS: Collimation
    VI. PITCH: Range specified
    VII. HELICAL EXPOSURE TIME: Single or multiple helix
    VIII. RECONSTRUCTION INTERVAL: Overlapping images
    IX. SUPERIOR AND INFERIOR EXTENT: Exam extent, orientation
    X. IV CONTRAST: Concentration, rate, scan delay, total volume
    XI. COMMENTS: Pertinent comments and ''pearls''

It is my hope that this book not only serve as a foundation for physicians performing helical CT, but that these protocols will be refined and adapted to each individual clinical practice.

Paul M. Silverman, M.D.

Acknowledgments

I would like to take this opportunity to thank my co-workers at Georgetown University Medical Center for all of their support and encouragement over the years. I also would like to thank the members of the Society of Computed Body Tomography and Magnetic Resonance (SCBT/MR) whose expertise and commitment to cross-sectional imaging at the highest level have set the gold standard. I would also like to acknowledge Keith Baldessari and Susan M. Garabedian-Ruffalo, PharmD. who first peaked my interest in developing a protocol book for both conventional and helical (spiral) CT. Finally, and most importantly, I want to thank all my co-authors: James A. Brink, M.D., Philip Costello, M.D., Elliott K. Fishman, M.D., Jay P. Heiken, M.D., Anthony A. Mancuso, M.D., David P. Naidich, M.D., Geoffrey D. Rubin, M.D., Ilona M. Schmalfuss, M.D., and Marilyn J. Siegel, M.D. for their dedication, hard work, and commitment to advancing the subspecialty of radiology by practicing the highest possible clinical care.

Helical (Spiral) Computed Tomography

A Practical Approach
To Clinical Protocols

Helical (Spiral) Computed Tomography,
edited by Paul M. Silverman.
Lippincott–Raven Publishers, Philadelphia © 1998.

1

Introduction to Principles and Clinical Practice of Helical (Spiral) CT Protocols

Paul M. Silverman

Division of Abdominal Imaging, Section of Computed Tomography, Georgetown University Medical Center, Washington, D.C. 20007

HISTORICAL CONSIDERATIONS

Since the clinical introduction of computed tomography (CT) in the mid-1970s, technical advances not only have improved image quality, but have dramatically altered the way in which such images are obtained. Conventional CT scanners incorporated complicated electrical cabling that coupled the x-ray tube and detector assembly to the reconstruction processor and high-voltage power supply. Individual scans were generally performed with a 2-sec scan time separated by a 6–7-sec interscan delay (ISD). The ISD was necessary to reorient the source-detector assembly within the gantry, preventing entanglement of the cables. The delay also allowed time for table movement and patient breathing between individual scans. The revolutionary development of a slip-ring gantry mechanism led to a new technology termed *helical*, or spiral, CT.

TECHNICAL CONSIDERATION OF HELICAL COMPUTED TOMOGRAPHY

Slip-ring technology consists of multiple sets of parallel rings and electrical components that rotate without constraint by cables. Data are assimilated by fixed brushes contacting multiple parallel rings. Voltage is supplied to the x-ray tube by a variety of mechanisms. Advanced detector technology is especially critical with helical CT, since the acquisition time is generally halved to 1 sec, limiting the total mAs that can be delivered. Some recent helical (spiral) scanners can even scan in the subsecond range. Standard older detectors with efficiencies on the order of 50% to 60% have generally been replaced with high-end, solid-state detectors with efficiencies in the range of 75% to 80%. One potential disadvantage of solid-state detectors, the afterglow phenomenon, has not been a clinical problem.

Generators and tubes must be more durable for helical CT. To deliver the high mAs of conventional scanning in one-half the time, generators and tubes for helical scanners must accommodate significant degrees of heat buildup and provide for the complexities of anode and focal tract cooling. The continued bombardment of the target with x-rays as occurs with helical CT produces extreme amounts of heat buildup in the anode. X-ray tubes with improved longevity are a focus of continued development.

With conventional CT, data are obtained from the same plane while the gantry rotates around a stationary patient. In contrast, with helical CT, the patient moves or is translated through the gantry as the helical data are obtained. This violates one of the fundamental requirements of conventional scanning, which is that CT reconstruction requires multiple views of precisely the same structures from at least 180 degrees plus the fan angle. Helical CT sections (except for those obtained by partial scans) are reconstructed from views taken over the 360-degree segment of the patient associated with one complete gantry rotation. Since the patient is continually moving through the gantry during the scan, no two data points are taken in exactly the same plane. After mathematical interpolation, the helical projection data are reconstructed, as they are with conventional scanning. The resulting helical image set is generally viewed as a series of conventional transaxial images or later processed employing software for multiplanar or three-dimensional imaging.

Before the initiation of a helical CT series, several scanning and reconstruction parameters must be specified. These parameters include collimation, table speed or incrementation, and image reconstruction interval. The ratio of the table speed or incrementation occurring during a complete tube rotation to the slice thickness is referred to as the helical ''pitch.'' This concept is new to CT technology. Figure 1 illustrates the relationship between pitch, table incrementation, and collimation.

$$\text{Pitch} = \frac{\text{Table Incrementation During Each Gantry Rotation}}{\text{Collimation}}$$

FIG. 1. Relationship between pitch, table incrementation, and collimation.

The scan coverage (Fig. 2) can be described as the product of the acquisition time and the table incrementation per gantry rotation period. The reconstruction length is shorter than the scan coverage because the first and last rotations of the x-ray tube are used to interpolate data at more central positions. Thus the reconstruction length is given by the product of the acquisition time less two gantry rotation periods and the table incrementation per gantry rotation period.

For example, a 1-cm collimation at a pitch ratio of 1.0(1:1) and a 30-sec helical exposure would cover 30 cm of tissue along the z-axis (e.g., the patient's torso). If a scan with a 2.0(2:1) pitch is desired, the table is set to move at a rate of two slice widths per second. The same 30-sec helix with 1-cm collimation will now cover 60 cm of tissue along the z-axis. Therefore the greater the helical pitch, the more coverage per breath-hold. In most helical CT studies a pitch of 1.0 will produce the best image quality. Increasing the helical pitch to greater than 1.0 increases the amount of anatomy covered during a designated scan time with a tradeoff in widening of the slice sensitivity profile (SSP) and more

Scan Coverage =

(Acquisition Time) x (Table Incrementation per Gantry Rotation Period)

Reconstruction Length =

(Acquisition Time - First and Last Gantry Rotation Periods)

x (Table Incrementation per Gantry Rotation Period)

FIG. 2. Definition of scan coverage and reconstruction length.

volume averaging. However, with current implementations of helical technology, the slice profile is widened in the range of 15% for a 1.5 pitch factor and routine scanning. This tradeoff may be applicable for more rapid screening of the abdomen or for such situations as when patients are uncooperative or ill. By increasing the table incrementation per gantry rotation using the same collimation, the volume of interest may be covered in a single breath-hold, which might be impossible in some patients using the standard 1.0 pitch. The use of increased pitch has been clearly beneficial in three-dimensional imaging since it allows for decreased collimation and resultant better image quality in the z-axis. Even in routine axial imaging, the tradeoff of increasing pitch may be beneficial to be able to decrease collimation. However, one may not be able to decrease the collimation significantly if image noise becomes unacceptable, especially in large patients or with scanners with significant tube current limitations. Modest increases in pitch are often effective in producing high quality without significant loss in clinical image quality. Generally a pitch of less than 2.0 is used.

CLINICAL ADVANTAGES OF HELICAL COMPUTED TOMOGRAPHY

There are many clinical, diagnostic, and patient-related advantages to helical CT technology. The chief advantage is the rapidity with which CT data are acquired. For example, almost the entire thorax may be helically scanned in a single 30-sec breath-hold; the same scan using conventional CT would require minutes. Single-breath-hold scan times may range from less than 10–15 sec to up to 30 sec. In general, individual breath-hold sequences usually range from 24 to 30 sec. In most cases if patients are coached appropriately and requested to practice hyperventilation prior to the examination, they can usually hold their breath for a full 30 sec. If the patient cannot hold his/her breath for this period, the exposure may be divided into two or three separate intervals, sometimes referred to as *double* or *triple helix scanning*. The rapid helical scanning process results in improved patient throughput, reduced scan times in individual patients, and completion of the scan before intravascular and interstitial concentrations of contrast material begin to equilibrate, maximizing vascular opacification and parenchymal lesion detectability.

Studies performed with conventional CT have shown the importance of rapid scanning after the administration of contrast media. In the liver, rapid scanning is critical, since lesions may become isodense with the hepatic parenchyma and difficult or even impossible to detect after contrast equilibration. The extremely rapid scanning possible with helical (spiral) CT can minimize such an effect but mandates the use of power injector for the consistent delivery of iodinated contrast media.

Additional clinical advantages of helical CT include improved lesion detection by eliminating respiratory misregistration and providing the new ability to reconstruct overlapping images at arbitrary intervals. Because helical scanning is performed during individual breath-holds, skips and overlaps resulting from variable inspirations during each individual scan as encountered with conventional step and shoot CT are eliminated. The acquisition of helical CT data without respiratory misregistration artifacts provides a quantum leap for improving the quality of two-dimensional and three-dimensional image reconstructions. The high-quality three-dimensional images that can be generated from helical data sets have dramatically changed the scope of this application in body CT. Historically, three-dimensional rendering with conventional CT was limited to bony structures because of their stationary nature and inherent high contrast differences from surrounding soft tissues. Vascular and soft-tissue three-dimensional renderings are much more complex and demanding because of overlapping or contiguous organs and the fact that pathologic processes may have similar attenuation values. Despite these challenges, helical CT has delivered excellent results. Commercially available sophisticated software packages now generate high-quality three-dimensional renderings of anatomic structures in the chest, abdomen, and pelvis. Advanced workstations have now brought CT imaging into the world of virtual reality, including virtual endoscopy and colonoscopy.

The ability to retrospectively shift the location of slice reconstruction is a major advantage of helical CT technology. Although the slice thickness or collimation is set before scan acquisition, the acquired raw data can be saved once reconstructed as image data. This can then be used to generate overlapping images (i.e., slice ''shift'' images) by any distance up to that of the original collimation. For example, if 10-mm collimation is used, slices may be reconstructed every 5 mm, 7 mm, or any other overlap, yielding a new set of images shifted in anatomic location. The ability to reconstruct images at arbitrarily chosen positions along the z-axis ensures that at least one of the images reconstructed is near the center of a lesion. The ability to reconstruct images at intervals smaller than the scan collimation reduces the possibility that a small lesion will be missed or not optimally characterized because of partial volume averaging. Overlapping images also provide additional images without any additional radiation exposure to the patient. Overlap of greater than 50% usually has diminished returns in general clinical practice but may be employed in specific cases to evaluate very small lesions.

LIMITATIONS OF HELICAL COMPUTED TOMOGRAPHY TECHNOLOGY

One of the minor disadvantages in performing helical CT scans of the abdomen, especially in the case of low-tier units, has been limitations in mAs, especially in large patients. In the case of these units, scan time may need to be increased from 1 to 1.5 sec. Most commercially available helical scanners use a technique of 120–140 kVp and 210–320 mAs to produce optimal-quality 7–10-mm slices. If a lower mA is used, the resulting images may be excessively grainy. If 3- or 5-mm collimation is used, a higher mA is often useful to produce scans that do not appear photogenic. Refinements in detector technology, higher-heat-capacity x-ray tubes, and other technical improvements will decrease limitations in achieving optimal image quality and anatomic coverage.

CLINICAL IMPACT

Since the introduction of helical CT in 1989 the technology has gained widespread clinical acceptance. Helical CT examinations have been used in studies of almost all areas of the body. It is expected that helical CT technology will eventually replace conventional CT. This book is designed to provide the user with an introduction to the technical features of helical scanning, a discussion of the background for establishing protocols, and a practical but detailed list of protocols to be used for helical CT examinations. The text is complemented by representative images that can be achieved when the protocols are employed.

CLINICAL APPLICATIONS OF HELICAL COMPUTED TOMOGRAPHY

Head and Neck Examinations

Helical CT of the head and neck offers several advantages over conventional CT examinations. One diagnostic advantage of the use of rapid scanning for head and neck studies is the reduction of artifacts caused by swallowing or respiratory motion. Most studies of the head and neck can be performed in one or two breath-holds. In selected situations some have suggested that amount of contrast material necessary to perform a helical scan series can be significantly reduced relative to conventional CT. Improved vascular opacification allows easier separation of nodes from vessels. Contrast enhancement of the primary head and neck tumor is also improved. High-quality three-dimensional and multiplanar images can be readily rendered. For example, when imaging the larynx, axial images can be supplemented by coronal or sagittal sections through areas of pathology to assist in surgical planning.

Helical CT, although in its infancy, shows great promise as a technology that is competitive with magnetic resonance imaging (MRI) and sonography in evaluating carotid artery stenosis. Unlike angiography, CT is both noninvasive and less expensive than MRI, and flow artifacts can often be avoided. It should be appreciated that multiple techniques of reconstruction evaluate different aspects of the vessels. Surface shaded display (SSD) images show the surface contour of vessels. This is analogous to reflecting a light off the surface of the image. The downside is that the internal architecture (i.e., plaques and atherosclerotic thrombi) cannot be characterized. Maximum-intensity projection (MIP) images allow the visualization of calcified plaques and are presently the most effective method of evaluating vascular stenosis. Other techniques under development will undoubtedly improve our ability to characterize carotid pathology. These three-dimensional techniques are specifically addressed in Chapter 7.

Chest Examinations

In thoracic imaging, helical CT is of major benefit since respiratory motion (i.e., misregistration, a common problem) is essentially eliminated. Helical CT is particularly useful when evaluating the lung bases where diaphragmatic motion on conventional CT may cause marked misregistration artifacts. Helical CT has been shown to be more effective in displaying normal anatomy and in detecting pulmonary nodules with the option of employing slice shifting.

The use of helical CT allows multiplanar and three-dimensional reconstruction of the thorax. These reconstructions are helpful in imaging the airways for tracheal tumors, tracheal stenosis, or bronchial dehiscence, and in evaluating the thoracic vasculature for aortic aneurysms and dissections. Since the volume of data can be reconstructed at thin increments through areas of suspected pathology, the airways can be exquisitely demonstrated by helical CT. However, this advantage may be negated if the original slice thickness is greater than the diameter of the lesion or if the pitch is significantly increased. For the most accurate densitometry, the section thickness should be one-half the diameter of the nodule.

Rapid helical scanning of the thorax allows the use of smaller volumes of contrast material than conventional CT. Studies have shown that the volume of contrast material necessary to enhance thoracic vascular structures can be reduced to approximately one-half that used for conventional dynamic incremental CT. Improved vascular opacification and image quality have even been demonstrated using 60 mL of 60% equivalent contrast media with helical technology, compared with 120 mL of contrast media required for conventional CT. Studies performed at the peak of contrast opacification facilitate detection of pulmonary emboli, vascular anomalies, and arteriovenous malformations. The role of helical CT in the diagnosis of pulmonary emboli is still evolving. To date, a number of studies have shown its effectiveness not only for central emboli but also for segmental emboli.

The approach to scanning the chest varies from institution to institution. The protocols provided allow for flexibility. Some institutions scan the chest rapidly after bolus initiation so that the liver is scanned well before equilibrium. Other institutions prefer to scan the liver first to time the upper abdominal study precisely and then to examine the chest. Excellent contrast enhancement of mediastinal vascular structures can still be achieved after liver scanning even with a 60–70-sec scan delay.

General Abdominal/Pelvic Examinations

Helical CT of the abdomen offers several advantages over conventional CT scanning. Helical CT of the abdomen and pelvis is best performed while the patient is in suspended expiration. Double or triple helix scanning may be necessary if the patient cannot hold his or her breath long enough to cover the entire area of interest.

Helical CT scanning of the abdomen is generally performed using a pitch of 1.0(1:1) to minimize blurring. In selective cases it may be helpful to use a pitch of greater than 1.0(1:1) (i.e., up to 2.0) to cover the entire volume of interest. Table 1 can be used to choose the appropriate table speed based on the reconstruction length needed for any helical examination. The following steps can be used to determine the collimation and table incrementation options for a given study. First, calculate from precontrast scans the image reconstruction length, which is needed to cover the volume of interest. Second, locate the appropriate reconstruction length on Table 1. The reconstruction lengths relate collimation and table incrementation options. For example, if a reconstruction length of 30 cm is needed, the table incrementation should be 10 mm for a 30-sec exposure and a pitch of 1.0(1:1). Sample collimation options are 5, 7, 8, or 10 mm, depending on the pitch used from 1.0(1:1) to 2.0(2:1). The user must keep in mind, however, that collimation options may vary from scanner to scanner. For most studies, reconstruction intervals equal to the slice thickness are sufficient. For the detection and characterization of small masses, overlapping reconstructions (i.e., reconstruction intervals smaller than the slice thickness) are useful. For multiplanar and three-dimensional reconstructions, very small reconstruction intervals provide the best detail.

As with conventional CT, rectal contrast media may be needed if oral contrast material does not opacify the rectosigmoid colon, if there is a pelvic mass, or if rectosigmoid pathology is suspected. In these cases, 150 mL of a dilute water-soluble agent (1% to 3%) is administered via an enema. In some cases, air may be substituted for a positive contrast agent. The use of a vaginal tampon may be helpful in adult female patients with suspected pelvic pathology.

Similar to conventional CT studies of the abdomen, oral contrast material is essential to distinguish a fluid-filled loop of bowel from a mass or abnormal fluid collection. A dilute barium suspension (1% to 2%) provides excellent bowel opacification, but a dilute water-soluble agent (2% to 4%) may alternatively be employed. A negative contrast agent (water)

TABLE 1. *Reconstruction length (cm) for pitch 1:1 to 2:1* (30-second exposure)*

Collimation (mm)	Table incrementation** (mm/sec)														
	2	3	4	5	6	7	8	9	10	11	12	13	14	15	16
2	6 (1.0)	9 (1.5)	12 (2.0)												
3		9 (1.0)	12 (1.3)	15 (1.7)	18 (2.0)										
5				15 (1.7)	18 (1.2)	21 (1.4)	24 (1.6)	27 (1.8)	30 (2.0)						
7						21 (1.0)	24 (1.1)	27 (1.3)	30 (1.4)	33 (1.6)	36 (1.7)	39 (1.9)	42 (2.0)		
8							24 (1.0)	27 (1.1)	30 (1.3)	33 (1.4)	36 (1.5)	39 (1.6)	42 (1.8)	45 (1.9)	48 (2.0)
10									30 (1.0)	33 (1.1)	36 (1.2)	39 (1.3)	42 (1.4)	45 (1.5)	48 (1.6)

* Pitch indicated in parentheses (pitch) has been rounded off.
** Table Incrementation = Table Speed (mm) in one rotation of the gantry (sec).

may also be useful to study the pancreas and upper abdominal vasculature and to eliminate artifacts that would otherwise compromise three-dimensional vascular reconstructions. Increasing the volume of oral contrast material administered provides greater bowel opacification. A minimum of 600 mL, but preferably 800–1000 mL, given 45–120 min before scanning, with an additional 200 mL ingested just prior to scanning, is recommended. A viscous oral contrast material can be used for evaluation of the esophagus. Patients who cannot drink the oral contrast material may require a nasogastric tube. In patients with bowel obstruction, the contrast material should be administered the night before the scheduled scan in order to achieve adequate bowel opacification.

The administration of intravenous (IV) contrast material during helical CT of the liver improves the detection and characterization of hepatic lesions. Radiologists agree that rapid scanning of the liver in the nonequilibrium phase is the preferred method for hepatic screening. Following the administration of IV contrast media at 2 mL/sec, peak liver enhancement has been reported approximately 120 sec after the initiation of the injection. Using a uniphasic injection technique, 70% of peak hepatic enhancement occurs after the termination of 150 mL of a 60% equivalent material bolus at rates of 2–3 mL/sec. Rapid helical CT of the liver offers a significant advantage over conventional CT in that the entire liver can be imaged during the time of peak contrast media enhancement. Even when using 7-mm collimation, the entire liver can be scanned in 30 sec in most patients. Some controversy remains concerning the appropriate delay between injection and scan initiation. Conventional CT scan delays of 21–45 sec are frequently recommended. We have found that with helical CT, optimal enhancement of the liver requires a longer delay, on the order of 60–75 sec, and depends on the rate of contrast injection. A disadvantage to the use of conventional CT in hepatic imaging is that current conventional scanners require approximately 1.5–2.5 min to complete an entire liver scan. Therefore unless, with the use of biphasic injection methodology, attention to technique is meticulous, a portion of the organ would be imaged during the contrast media equilibrium phase, when it may be more likely to overlook lesions. The very brief scan time of helical CT allows for considerable flexibility in hepatic scanning. Scanning during the optimal temporal window can now be achieved more closely. New Computer Automated Scanning Technology (CAST) has proven effective in not only providing improved contrast enhancement of the liver, but in increasing consistency from patient to patient. This approach can allow equivalent quality examination of the liver using less intravenous contrast. In addition, multiple passes can be utilized to study the liver in different vascular phases to improve the detectability of hypervascular hepatic tumors (e.g., hepatoma, neuroendocrine tumors, renal cell carcinoma, breast carcinoma, metastatic melanoma, and sarcoma). Early first-pass scanning at 15–20 sec will optimally detect hypervascular metastases followed by complimentary scanning during the portal venous phase, 60–70 sec. For optimal results, rates of contrast injection should be in the range of 4–6 mL/sec.

Included in the protocols is the title reconstruction interval, referring to overlapping images. Most physicians elect to film just the routine slices and only view selectively reconstructed overlapping slices when there is a question, since filming of all images is expensive and time-consuming. It has been demonstrated that for either detection or characterization of small lesions in the liver, it may be useful to reconstruct 7–10-mm-thick slices every 4 or 5 mm to compensate for partial volume averaging.

The advent of helical CT may improve our ability to image pancreatic carcinomas. Although contrast media dynamics in the pancreas are not as well defined as those for the liver, it is clear that these tumors are best visualized when the circulating levels of contrast are high and dual-phase imaging is useful with an initial acquisition during the pancreatic phase, beginning 30 sec after initiation of the contrast injection. The hepatic phase can begin immediately after the conclusion of the pancreatic phase. In addition, the ability to shift the reconstructed slice locations permits visualization of small or subtle pancreatic lesions. The speed of helical CT is advantageous because the entire pancreas can be imaged while the circulating level of contrast material is high (i.e., nonequilibrium phase). Vascular involvement in pancreatic carcinoma is better displayed with both axial and three-dimensional helical CT and is of great clinical importance in determining surgical resectability.

Helical CT scanning of the pancreas can be performed from head to foot or from foot to head. When scanning from below (foot to head), thin (5-mm) sections of the pancreas are followed by hepatic imaging. Although this technique can be completed during the nonequilibrium phase of the contrast material, a potential pitfall is that the superior mesenteric vein may not be optimally opacified. Scanning in the head-to-foot direction may miss the uncinate portion of the pancreas unless careful attention is made in the protocol as to the extent of the thin-section slices. Precontrast scans can be useful in this case to set up the extent of the thin-section helical scan series through the pancreas.

Helical CT of the kidneys provides for rapid scanning without respiratory misregistration and is excellent for visualizing renal parenchymal tissue and renal vasculature. As with other organs, the ability to perform retrospective reconstructions at overlapping intervals improves the detectability of small lesions. Rescanning may be helpful, since in the beginning of the bolus phase (i.e., the corticomedullary phase), the medullary portion of the kidneys is not enhanced and lesions in this area of the kidney may be missed. Rescanning after the medullary portion opacifies, the nephrogram phase complements interpretation. Delayed images during the excretory phase allow one to distinguish parapelvic cysts from hydronephrosis. In patients with renal cell carcinoma, arterial tumor vascularity and renal vein invasion are readily assessed. Three-dimensional imaging also provides great promise in assessing for renal artery stenosis. Another new application for helical CT is the detection of ureteral calculi. In this situation, helical CT without contrast is employed to detect ureteral stones, obviating the need for a potentially more time-consuming intravenous urogram.

Musculoskeletal/Bone Examinations

Helical CT examinations have had an impact in the musculoskeletal area, especially in the area of bone pathology, particularly tumors and musculoskeletal tumors. The ability of helical CT to rapidly assess the integrity of both the soft tissues and the bones in the case of extensive blunt trauma has made it highly cost effective. Magnetic resonance imaging (MRI) remains the test of choice for joint disorders. With the development of more advanced computer hardware and software, striking displays of bone pathology can be effectively conveyed to our clinical colleagues to assist in planning surgical intervention.

Pediatric Examinations

Helical CT provides a number of distinct advantages over conventional CT in the pediatric age group, the most important of which is the rapid scanning speed critical for optimal patient cooperation. Within the section on pediatric imaging a detailed discussion includes the approach to sedation. Also included are guidelines for dosages of oral contrast stratified to age and, most important, total volume, rate of administration of iodinated contrast material, and needle size matched to the injection rate. Technical parameters—including the slice thickness, pitch, and extent of breath-hold—are clearly outlined to facilitate each examination protocol. The valuable guidelines in the chapter on pediatric helical CT (Chapter 6) complemented by the detailed protocols are exceptionally valuable to those radiologists who do not routinely scan patients in the pediatric age group. The protocols are tailored to the most likely clinical problems, and pitfalls of helical CT are addressed. All anatomic areas are addressed to ensure the highest-quality clinical examinations.

Three-Dimensional Examinations

Since helical CT is a volumetric data acquisition, three-dimensional imaging of vascular and soft tissues has become a reality. Chapter 7 and its protocols provide a comprehensive approach to optimizing the parameters used to acquire the data to create the best images. Discussions of contrast techniques, reconstruction approaches, and rendering and editing of data provide the basic principles needed for practicing radiologists. The protocols clearly describe the approach needed to produce high-quality three-dimensional images.

SUMMARY

Helical acquisition of CT data has rapidly become state of the art in radiology. The increased scanning speed provides improved parenchymal and vascular opacification despite the use of less contrast in many clinical applications. Additionally, the ability to do three-dimensional imaging is a major advantage over prior conventional technology.

SUGGESTED READING

Beregi J, Elkohen M, Deklunder G, Artaud D, Coullet JM, Wattinne L. Helical CT angiography compared with arteriography in the detection of renal artery stenosis. *AJR* 1996;167:495–501.

Birnbaum BA, Jacobs JE, Yin D. Hepatic enhancement during helical CT: a comparison of moderate rate uniphasic and biphasic contrast injection protocols. *AJR* 1995;165:853–858.

Bluemke DA, Fishman EK. Spiral CT of the liver. *AJR* 1992;160:787–792.

Bonaldi VM, Bret PM, Reinhold C, Mostafa, A. Helical CT of the liver: value of an early hepatic arterial phase. *Radiology* 1995;197:357–363.

Brink JA. Technical aspects of helical (spiral) CT. *Radiol Clin North Am* 1995;33:825–841.

Brink JA, Heiken JP, Forman HP, Sagel SS, Molina PL, Brown PC. Hepatic spiral CT: reduction of dose of intravenous contrast material. *Radiology* 1995;197:83–88.

Cohan RH, Sherman LS, Korobkin M, Bass JC, Francis IR. Renal masses: assessment of corticomedullary-phase and nephrographic-phase CT scans. *Radiology* 1991;196:445–451.

Costello P, Anderson W, Blume D. Pulmonary nodule: evaluation with spiral volumetric CT. *Radiology* 1991;179: 875–876.

Costello P, Dupuy DE, Ecker CP, Tello R. Spiral CT of the thorax with reduced volume of contrast material: a comparative study. *Radiology* 1992;193:663–666.

Costello P, Ecker CP, Tello R, Hartnell GG. Assessment of the thoracic aorta by spiral CT. *AJR* 1992;158:1127–1130.

Diedrichs CG, Keating DP, Glatting G, Oestmann JW. Blurring of vessels in spiral CT angiography: effects of collimation width, pitch, viewing plane and windowing in maximum intensity projection. *J Comput Assist Tomogr* 1996;20(6):965–974.

Dupuy DE, Costello P, Ecker CP. Spiral CT of the pancreas. *Radiology* 1992;183:815–818.

Fishman EK. Spiral CT evaluation of the musculoskeletal system. In: Fishman EK, Jeffrey RB, eds., *Spiral CT: principles, techniques and clinical application*. New York: Raven Press, 1995;141–158.

Foley WD. Dynamic hepatic CT. *Radiology* 1989;170:617–622.

Freeny PC, Gardner JC, vonlngersleben G, Heyano S, Nghiem HV, Winter TC. Hepatic helical CT: effect of reduction of iodine dose of intravenous contrast material on hepatic contrast enhancement. *Radiology* 1995;197:89–93.

Galanski M, Prokop M, Chavan A, Schaefer CM, Jandeleit K, Nischelsky JE. Renal arterial stenoses: spiral CT angiography. *Radiology* 1993;189:185–192.

Heiken JP, Brink JA, McClennan BL, et al. Dynamic contrast-enhanced CT of the liver: comparison of contrast medium injection rates and uniphasic and biphasic injection protocols. *Radiology* 1993;187:327–331.

Heiken JP, Brink JA, McClennan BL, Sagel SS, Crowe TM, Gains MV. Dynamic incremental CT: effect of volume and concentration of contrast material and patient weight on hepatic enhancement. *Radiology* 1995;195:353–357.

Heiken JP, Brink JA, Vannier MW. Spiral (helical) CT. *Radiology* 1993;189:647–656.

Ibukuro K, Charnsangavej C, Chasen MH, et al. Helical CT angiography with multiplanar reformation: techniques and clinical applications. *Radiographics* 1995;15(3):671–682.

Johnson PT, Heath DG, Kuszyk BS, Fishman EK. CT angiography with volume rendering: advantages and applications in splanchnic vascular imaging. *Radiology* 1996;200(2):564–568.

Kalender WA, Seissler W, Klotz E, et al. Spiral volumetric CT with single-breath-hold technique, continuous transport, and continuous scanner rotation. *Radiology* 1990;176:181–183.

Lu DSK, Vendantham S, Krasny RM, Kadell B, Berger WL, Reber HA. Two-phase helical CT for pancreatic tumor: pancreatic versus hepatic phase enhancement of tumor, pancreas and vascular structures. *Radiology* 1996;199: 697–701.

Marks MP, Napel S, Jordan JE, Enzmann DR. Diagnosis of carotid artery disease: preliminary experience with maximum-intensity-projection spiral CT angiography. *AJR* 1993;160:1267–1271.

McEnery KW, Wilson AJ, Murphy WA Jr, Marushack MM. Spiral CT imaging of the musculoskeletal system: a phantom study. *Radiology* 1992;185(P):118.

Napel S, Marks MP, Rubin GD, et al. CT angiography with spiral CT and maximum intensity projection. *Radiology* 1992;185(2):607–610.

Ney DR, Fishman EK, Kawashima A, et al. Comparison of helical and spiral CT with regard to three-dimensional imaging of musculoskeletal anatomy. *Radiology* 1992;185:865–869.

Ney DR, Fishman EK, Kawashima A, Robertson DD Jr, Scott WW. Comparison of helical and serial CT with regard to three-dimensional imaging of musculoskeletal anatomy. *Radiology* 1992;185:865–869.

Polacin A, Kalender WA, Marchal C. Evaluation of section sensitivity profiles and image noise in spiral CT. *Radiology* 1992;185:29–35.

Pretorius ES, Fishman EK. Helical (spiral) CT of the musculoskeletal system. *Radiol Clin North Am* 1995;33(5): 949–979.

Raptopoulos V, Rosen MP, Kent KC, Kuestner LM, Sheiman RG, Pearlman JD. Sequential helical CT angiography of aortoiliac disease. *AJR* 1996;166:1347–1354.

Remy J, Reny-Jaron M, Giraud F, Wattinne L. Angioarchitecture of pulmonary arteriovenous malformation: clinical utility of three-dimensional helical CT. *Radiology* 1994;191:657–664.

Remy-Jardin M, Remy J, Deschildre F, et al. Diagnosis of pulmonary embolism with spiral CT: comparison with pulmonary angiography and scintigraphy. *Radiology* 1996;200:699–706.

Rubin GD, Lane M, Bloch D, Leung AU, Stark P. Optimizing of thoracic spiral CT: effects of iodinated contrast medium concentration. *Radiology* 1996;201:785–791.

Rubin GD, Dake MD, Napel SA, et al. Spiral CT of renal artery stenosis: comparison of three-dimensional rendering techniques. *Radiology* 1994;190:181–189.

Rubin GD, Dake MD, Napel S, et al. Spiral CT of renal artery stenosis: comparison of three-dimensional rendering techniques. *Radiology* 1994;190:181–189.

Schwartz RB, Jones KM, Chenoff DM, et al. Common carotid artery bifurcation: evaluation with spiral CT. *Radiology* 1992;185:513–519.

Silverman PM, Cooper C, Zeman RK, Garra BS, Trock B, Davros WJ. Establishing the optimal window for liver CT using a time density analysis: implications for helical CT. *J Comput Assist Tomogr* 1995;19(1):73–79.

Silverman PM, Cooper C, Zeman RK. Imaging of the liver: a survey update of prevailing techniques for conventional CT scanning. *Abdom Imaging* 1995;20(4):348–352.

Silverman PM and Korobkin M: High resolution computed tomography of the normal larynx. *AJR* 1983;140:875–880.

Silverman PM, O'Malley J, Cooper C, Zeman RK, Tefft MC. Detection of hepatic metastases by helical (spiral) CT: optimizing of timing after contrast administration for assess the conspicuity of metastatic disease. *AJR* 1995; 164:619–623.

Silverman PM, Roberts SC, Ducic I, et al. Assessment of a technology that permits individualized scan delays in helical hepatic CT: a technique to improve efficiency in the use of contrast material. *AJR* 1996;167:79–84.

Silverman SG, Lee BY, Seltzer SE, Bloom DA, Corless CL, Adams DF. Small (less than 3 cm) renal masses: correlation of spiral CT features and pathologic findings. *AJR* 1994;163:597–605.

Urban BA, Fishman EK, Kuhlman JE, Kawashima A, Hennessey JG, Siegelman SS. Detection of focal hepatic lesions with spiral CT: comparison of 4- and 8-mm interscan spacing. *AJR* 1993;160:783–785.

Van Hoe L, Baert AL, Gryspeerdt S, et al. Supra- and juxtarenal aneurysms of the abdominal aorta: preoperative assessment with thin section spiral CT. *Radiology* 1996;198:443–448.

Walkey MM. Dynamic hepatic CT: how many years will it take til we learn? *Radiology* 1991;181:17–24.

Winter TC, Nghiem HV, Schmiedl UP, Freeny PC. CT angiography of the visceral vessels. *Semin Ultrasound CT MR.* 1996;17(4):339–352.

Zeman RK, Fox SH, Silverman PM, et al. Helical (spiral) CT of the abdomen. *AJR* 1993;160:719–725.

Zeman RK, Zeiberg AS, Davros WJ, et al. Routine helical CT of the abdomen: image quality considerations. *Radiology* 1993;189:395–400.

Helical (Spiral) Computed Tomography,
edited by Paul M. Silverman.
Lippincott–Raven Publishers, Philadelphia © 1998.

2

Protocols for Helical CT of the Head and Neck

Ilona M. Schmalfuss and Anthony A. Mancuso

Department of Radiology, University of Florida, College of Medicine, Gainesville, Florida 32610

It is widely accepted that helical computed tomography (CT), with its rapid data acquisition, reduces, if not eliminates, motion artifacts such as respiratory misregistration seen with conventional CT (1). This aspect of helical CT alone is important in imaging of the head and neck region. Swallowing artifacts in particular can cause clinically significant degradation of images in studies of the oropharynx, larynx, and hypopharynx (Fig. 1). Respiratory motion may produce gaps in the scanned area, a difficulty most commonly encountered in the larynx (2).

The markedly reduced motion artifacts with helical CT can also reduce the need for sedation, especially in pediatric patients. Sedation may still be required with subsequent three-dimensional reconstruction of the region of critical interest, as in patients with craniosynostosis or craniofacial malformation, which sometimes require thin sections. Any motion during scanning of these patients can result in a nondiagnostic study that will then be repeated and result in additional radiation exposure (3). The major advance that comes with helical data acquisition is the flexibility with which the data set can be reconstructed. In general, intravenous contrast is used more effectively with helical technique, but reduction in the volume of contrast used has been modest.

There is only a small price to pay in terms of spatial and contrast resolution when helical data acquisition is used, and it seems insignificant in the head and neck region. Only beam hardening and resultant degradation of images through the shoulder region remain insoluble problems with the current tube/detector system.

IMAGING TECHNIQUE

Gantry Angle

In general, the gantry angles using helical CT technique are the same as those in conventional CT. The head and the portions of the neck and face cephalad to the hard palate are scanned with the gantry angled parallel to the inferior orbital meatal line (IOML). The remainder of the neck and pharynx is studied with the gantry angled parallel to the body of the mandible (Fig. 2). Slightly modified angulation of the gantry around the teeth is sometimes necessary to avoid artifacts from dental amalgam and to ensure coverage of the entire oropharynx and majority of the oral cavity without dental artifacts. The coronal scan plane is made as perpendicular to the IOML as possible (4).

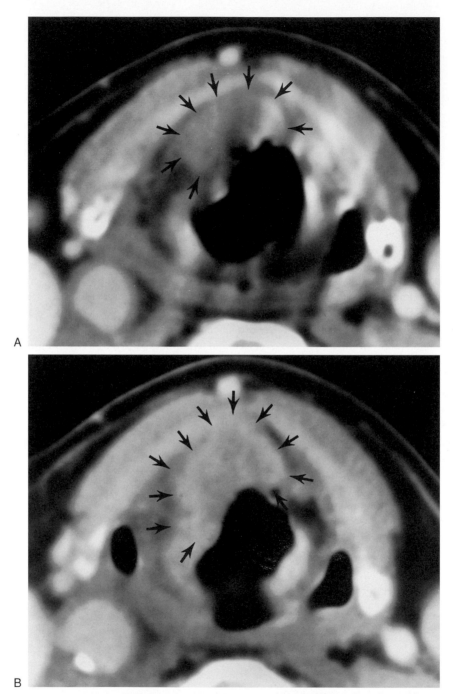

FIG. 1. (**A**) The extent of the supraglottic cancer (*arrows*) is difficult to determine on the image obtained with conventional technique using 3-mm slice thickness and spacing secondary to degradation by motion artifacts. (**B**) No motion artifacts or blurring are present on this helical CT image obtained at approximately the same level and same day with 3-mm slice thickness and a pitch of 1.4. The tumor size and extent can be easier demarcated (*arrows*).

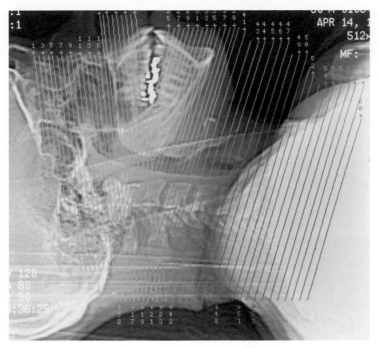

FIG. 2. The lateral scout of the neck demonstrates the different angulation of the CT images around the teeth to minimize artifacts caused by dental fillings. The overlapping of the images in the oropharynx ascertains coverage of the entire oropharynx without dental artifacts.

There are some exceptions to these general rules. The examination of the larynx, for example, requires scanning with the gantry angled parallel to the true vocal cords to avoid distortion of anatomic landmarks critical for treatment planning (Fig. 3A). Inaccurate gantry angle can cause artificial ''thickening'' of the anterior commissure, indicating more extensive disease in patients with laryngeal tumors than is actually present (Fig. 3B). Partial volume averaging of the true or false vocal cords with the interposed laryngeal ventricle (Fig. 3C) may result in inability to evaluate the paraglottic fat planes that play a key role in determination of the deep extension, and therefore surgical approach, of some laryngeal cancers. Occasionally, the obliteration of these fat planes is the only sign that a lesion is present at all (5).

Whenever reformation in the coronal or sagittal plane as well as three-dimensional reconstructions are considered, the gantry should remain in neutral (0-degree angle) position to allow faster data processing. In general, reformations are possible from axial images obtained with tilted gantry, but the data processing requires more sophisticated computer software and significantly more time. So far, there are no results that compare the imaging quality and anatomic detail of reformations performed in coronal and/or sagittal plane from a set of axial images obtained with off 0-degree gantry angles. Only limited published results are available in this regard for three-dimensional reconstructions in the head and neck region (6). This study shows that most readers preferred a gantry tilt of −30 degrees (parallel to the facet joints) for the evaluation of three-dimensional images of the spine because of better depiction of joint spaces; however, the actual quality of three-dimensional images reconstructed from axial acquisitions with gantry tilts was not significantly different from that with no gantry angulation (6). It is uncertain if these results are applicable to other areas of the head and neck. Axial images for subsequent reformations in coronal and/or sagittal plane and those

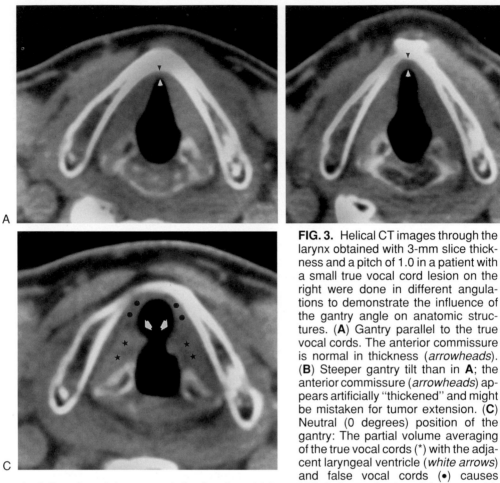

FIG. 3. Helical CT images through the larynx obtained with 3-mm slice thickness and a pitch of 1.0 in a patient with a small true vocal cord lesion on the right were done in different angulations to demonstrate the influence of the gantry angle on anatomic structures. (**A**) Gantry parallel to the true vocal cords. The anterior commissure is normal in thickness (*arrowheads*). (**B**) Steeper gantry tilt than in **A**; the anterior commissure (*arrowheads*) appears artificially "thickened" and might be mistaken for tumor extension. (**C**) Neutral (0 degrees) position of the gantry: The partial volume averaging of the true vocal cords (*) with the adjacent laryngeal ventricle (*white arrows*) and false vocal cords (•) causes marked distortion of the anatomic landmarks, which could limit the evaluation of this area with regard to planning the suitability of a lesion for voice conservation surgery. It is important to note that in helical CT, axial reformations parallel to the true vocal cords can also be obtained retrospectively if the scan was obtained with an inappropriate gantry angle.

used for three-dimensional reconstruction are made with 0-degree gantry tilt with the head positioned so that the hard palate is aligned as parallel as possible to the gantry angle.

Contrast

With the introduction of helical CT and its rapid data acquisition it was thought that the intravenous contrast would decrease dramatically. Spreer and colleagues compared the enhancement of the main vasculature of the neck as well as that of various soft-tissue structures on conventional CT scans with those done with helical technique (7). They found that a contrast dose reduced by one-third resulted in the same or even better enhancement of the main vessels of the neck using helical CT imaging. The enhancement of the soft tissues was similar in the two techniques in the upper neck but less intense in the lower neck using helical CT (7). These results are not confirmed in our practice, where the dose of contrast used in the average study has not been reduced. Perhaps the discrepancy between our practice and the result of Spreer is related to differences in scan protocols. The protocol of Spreer and colleagues covered the entire neck using 5-mm collimation and no apparent angulation around the teeth. Five-millimeter-slice thickness is insufficient for almost all head and neck regions, and alterations of gantry angulation during scanning are a must for consistently meaningful studies. Because of this, an adequate CT evaluation typically requires a minimum of two acquisition sets when the entire neck is scanned with angulation in between the acquisitions. This requires longer scanning times and higher contrast doses than those proposed by Spreer.

In general, 150 mL of intravenous contrast is necessary if angulation of the gantry is required and 100 mL if not. The dose is adjusted for pediatric patients. Forty-five milliliters of contrast is injected at 1 mL/sec prior to the scan (i.e., a 45-sec scan delay) followed by infusion of the remaining volume at a rate of 0.5 mL/sec. For routine brain studies the injection rate is 0.5 mL/sec with scanning beginning after a 5-min delay. Evaluation of the extracranial and intracranial vessels requires an injection rate of 3 mL/sec with a 20-sec scan delay.

Slice Thickness/Collimation

In general, the best image quality is obtained when the reconstruction interval is equal to the slice thickness or when the reconstructions are performed with overlapping slices (3). For example, the original data set obtained with 3-mm collimation can be reconstructed into images of same-slice thickness, but in 1-mm increments only resulting in 2-mm overlap of adjacent images (Figs. 4 and 5). A very small reconstruction interval (e.g., 0.2 mm in temporal bone) without and with overlapping slices is possible but not necessarily practical because of the higher number of images to be reviewed which require longer data-processing time and larger storage space (8).

The basic slice thickness (collimation) for the different head and neck areas is as follows:

- Head: 3 mm through the posterior fossa, 5 and 7 mm through the remainder of the head in children and adults, respectively.
- Facial bones, neck, orbit, and sinuses: 3 mm; if direct coronal imaging of the facial bones, orbit, or sinuses is impossible, the axial images are obtained with 1-mm-slice thickness to improve the quality of reformations.
- Temporal bone: 1 mm.

Adjustment of the slice thickness may be required for certain indications (see specific protocols).

Pitch

The pitch is directly proportional to slice broadening, and increasing pitch thereby directly diminishes longitudinal resolution; therefore a pitch of 1 is considered optimal for preserving the z-axis resolution. Realistically, there is a tradeoff between scanning time, coverage length, radiation to the patient, and image quality. A pitch of up to 1.5 is almost always adequate for evaluating the head and neck region. With this pitch choice, the slice profile is widened to a maximum of 15%. A pitch of 1 is required only when multiplanar *reformations* of very small anatomic structures (e.g., ossicles, cribriform plate) are required for accurate diagnosis.

Tube Current

The tube current (mAs) is a critical factor in helical CT imaging. In areas of high inherent contrast such as the sinuses, facial bones, temporal bone, and even extracranial soft tissues,

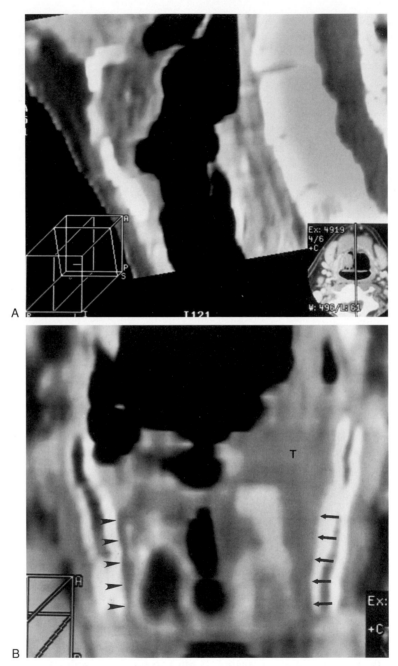

FIG. 4. Sagittal (**A**) and coronal (**B**) reformations performed from axial images of a helical CT scan obtained with 3-mm slice thickness and a pitch of 1.0 without overlapping of the slices. The images are of slightly superior quality to reformations from conventional CT (not shown). The coronal image demonstrates the laryngeal tumor on the left (T), which was extending superiorly to the vallecula and inferiorly to the true vocal cord. The inferior extent is best appreciated when the paraglottic fat planes (*arrowheads*) are evaluated. These are well visualized on the right (*arrowheads*) and are completely obliterated on the left (*small arrows*).

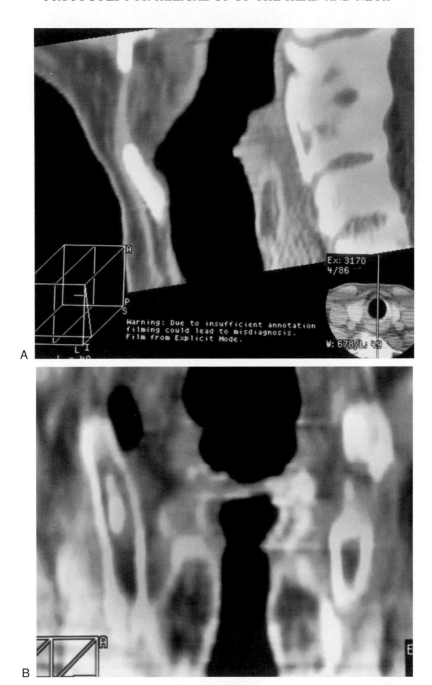

FIG. 5. Sagittal (**A**) and coronal (**B**) reformations of the larynx demonstrate improved quality of the reformations in comparison with Fig. 4. The axial images were acquired with the same technique and parameters (3-mm slice thickness, pitch 1.0) as in Fig. 4, but the reformations were obtained with 2-mm overlap between adjacent axial slices (i.e., from an axial set of images reconstructed at 1-mm increments).

a current of 200–250 mAs is usually sufficient for excellent image quality. For the studies focusing on structures with low inherent contrast, such as brain, the maximal possible current is applied except in pediatric patients. Even the maximal technique may result in suboptimal demonstration of the soft tissues, with increased noise, poor contrast, and grainy images. This is most apparent in studies of the brain and those of the neck when the scan extends far enough inferiorly to require imaging through the shoulders. These shoulder artifacts are particularly troublesome, and conventional techniques through the shoulder at 120 kV and 300 mA/2 sec are used to optimize the image quality. Motion artifacts are not common at the shoulder level, so that helical data acquisition is not as important in this region as it is in the sections through the mid-pharynx. Children and adults with smaller body habitus are exceptions to this problem.

DATA RECONSTRUCTION AND REFORMATION

Reconstruction

In volumetric CT the movement of the radiation through the subject occurs in a helical fashion, and the acquired data are never from exactly the same plane. Complex mathematical interpolation is necessary to reconstruct these data into images. This process has certain advantages over conventional CT but also some limitations.

Slice Thickness

In contrast to conventional CT, helical CT as a volumetric acquisition technique allows retrospective reconstruction of the data at any interval without increasing the scanning time or radiation to the patient (see also the earlier discussion). Therefore the slice thickness used during scanning does not have to be equal to the slice thickness of subsequently reconstructed and displayed images.

Slice Overlapping

Reconstructions can also be obtained with variable slice overlapping, which can improve the anatomic detail in certain areas. This is of special interest in the temporal bone, where very small structures are imaged and conventional CT technique may be limited in regard to slice thickness and its resolution capacity. The added radiation dose that would result from overlapping slices cannot be justified. For certain indications, such as congenital hearing loss, 0.5-mm reconstruction intervals are used for helical CT images made with 1-mm collimation through the temporal bone. This allows more definitive visualization of the inner ear structures and the ossicles, especially the footplate of the stapes, the modiolus, and the vestibular aqueduct. So far, only limited published results are available with regard to the use of high-resolution overlapped sections (9). This group reports that in general the in-plane spatial resolution of the helical CT is similar to conventional CT. Using helical technique, it found better demonstration of the footplate of the stapes with overlapping images but diminished visualization of the stapes superstructure in one patient with middle ear opacification following trauma when conventional and helical techniques are compared. The group considered the lower contrast of helical CT as a possible reason (9). The use of higher mAs suggested in the protocols in this chapter should overcome this effect.

Contrast Resolution

Examinations of phantoms show the visibility of low-contrast lesions to be reduced on helical CT because of increased image noise and increased slice sensitivity profile compared with conventional CT (1). These two factors are apparently more noticeable in imaging of small soft-tissue structures with thinner sections, such as in the head and neck region, than of larger soft-tissue structures scanned with thicker sections. In addition, the elongation of the slice sensitivity profile in helical CT as a volumetric acquisition increases partial volume effect, which may reduce the detection of small lesions, especially if these are of low inherent contrast with the surrounding normal tissue (1). One group suggests that these theoretical results obtained on phantoms support the results of studies on patients having head and neck CT examinations, which showed decreased detection of subtle, relatively low-contrast abnormalities. In particular, this group noted decreased visualization of the paraglottic fat planes on helical CT in comparison with conventional technique; the obliteration of these planes may be the only sign of an underlying lesion or can cause underestimation of the extent of the laryngeal tumor (1). This theoretical fault, however, has not resulted in practical problems in our day-to-day evaluation of patients with laryngeal carcinoma, where helical techniques are used routinely in the larynx.

Reformation

Coronal and sagittal reformations are used mainly as a default technique in patients who cannot tolerate the position for direct coronal imaging and when the sagittal plane might add important information related to the planning of treatment. Reformations may also be used to avoid artifacts from dental amalgam (10). Multiplanar reformations using the helical technique are consistently better quality than those done with conventional CT because of the apparent reduction of volume averaging between sections in the z-axis (see Figs. 4 and 5).

Nevertheless, even reformations from helical CT are suboptimal in comparison with direct coronal imaging. In regions where thin bone lies within the imaging axial plane, reformations of the axial data set may lead to mistaking the thin bone for bone loss or dehiscence on the reformatted images. One group has reported that this is clearly a pitfall of helical CT wherein the tegmen of the middle ear, the cortical margin of the tympanic facial canal (Fig. 6) and fine ethmoidal septations, and the cribriform plate (Fig. 7) may appear dehiscent (9). This is a particularly important limitation in patients with CSF leakage where CT must often detect very subtle areas of dehiscence or discontinuity in the skull base. Direct coronal imaging is preferred whenever possible in such situations (Fig. 8).

Three-Dimensional Display

Three-dimensional display is used most often in evaluating craniofacial abnormalities such as craniosynostosis and facial fractures. It has also been used sparingly for the study of laryngeal or subglottic stenosis, integrity of the ossicular chain, spinal abnormalities, and determination of tumor volume. Three-dimensional display is used mainly as an aid in planning surgery rather than for diagnosis. Helical CT produces higher-quality three-dimensional images than conventional CT. The image quality can be improved even more by using thinner slices and larger slice overlap (3). The region of interest might not be covered with *one* helical acquisition; consequently, multiple acquisitions may be obtained in series to complete the study. Artifacts on three-dimensional reformations caused by suboptimal technique in the head region have been described (3). These include:

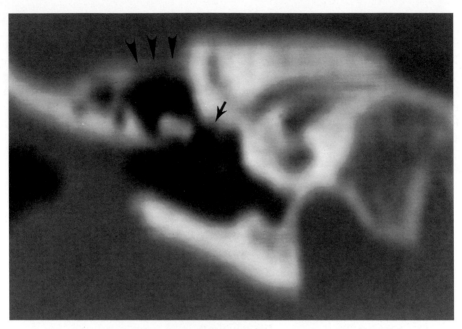

FIG. 6. This coronal reformation was obtained from axial images of a helical CT scan acquired with 1-mm slice thickness, 1.0-mm pitch, and 0.5-mm overlap of the axial slices. It demonstrates superior anatomic detail to conventional reformations (not shown), but the roof of the middle ear (*arrowheads*) and the tympanic portion of the facial canal (*arrow*) remain a problematic area where normally thin bone may appear dehiscent on the reformatted images.

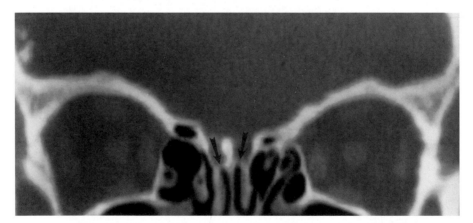

FIG. 7. This coronal reformation was performed from axial images of a helical CT scan obtained with 1-mm slice thickness and a pitch of 1.4. It demonstrates small gaps (*arrows*) bilaterally in a patient with an intact cribriform plate. This area might be incorrectly interpreted as dehiscence in a patient with CSF rhinorrhea.

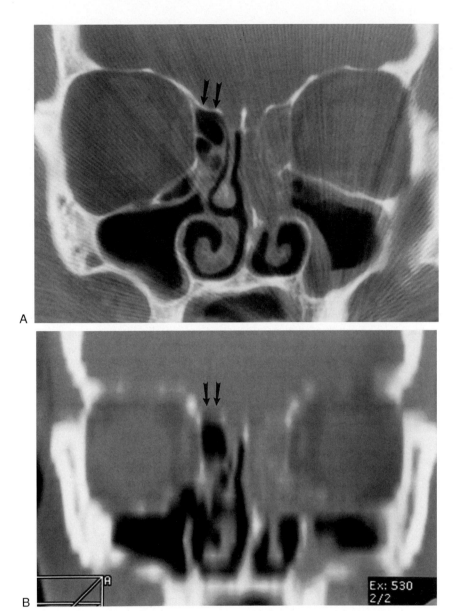

FIG. 8. Direct coronal image (**A**) through the sinuses and nasal cavity obtained in helical technique (3-mm slice thickness, 1.4 pitch) is slightly degraded by artifacts caused by dental fillings on the left. This can be especially problematic in patients with a large number of dental fillings. In these patients, coronal reformations from axial images can entirely avoid the type of image degradation as seen in **B**. (**B**) This reformatted image in coronal plane is of lower anatomic detail than the direct coronal image (e.g., the roof of the ethmoid air cells on the right appears dehiscent (*arrows* in [B]) in contrast to the direct coronal scan (*arrows* in **A**)). The anatomic detail can be significantly improved if the axial images are acquired with 1-mm-slice thickness and a pitch of less than 1.5 (see also Fig. 7) or if the reformations are performed with overlapping axial slices (see also sinuses/nasal cavity protocol without iv contrast). In general, direct coronal scanning is recommended; however, helical techniques of appropriate resolving power can be substituted if the patient cannot tolerate direct coronal imaging.

- *Chainsaw artifact.* This artifact occurs when data of few slices are missing, which typically is seen between the adjacent helical acquisition sets. This problem can be solved by overlapping the end and start of these acquisitions.
- *Boiled egg artifact.* This artifact occurs in the high parietal region when data are missing through the last few millimeters of the head. This can be avoided by coverage of the head beyond the vertex.
- *Distortion.* Distortion of the shape of the head on the three-dimensional display can occur when the available software cannot compensate for the gantry tilt. This can be eliminated by scanning in neutral position (gantry angle of 0 degrees).
- *Lego effect.* The Lego effect is caused by squared edges of each slice at the convexity. This artifact can be overcome by using the smoothing algorithm during three-dimensional reconstructions or thinner slice thickness, preferably 1 mm, during scanning.
- *Threshold selection.* The three-dimensional image appearance is dependent on the chosen threshold during reconstructions. For instance, increasing the value will open sutures and enlarge pseudo-foramina; decreasing the threshold will mistakenly close the sutures.

Some of these artifacts also occur in other regions in the head and neck.

Three-dimensional reformations of the larynx, subglottic region, and hypopharynx can provide an endoscopic view through this region and supplement the diagnostic endoscopic examination (11,12). Such three-dimensional images nicely display the areas of luminal narrowing as an airway cast and are therefore complementary to the cross-sectional images. The three-dimensional display does not demonstrate the adjacent soft tissues (11). One group evaluating the value of such postprocessing showed that otolaryngologists ranked the three-dimensional images as more beneficial than radiologists did, usually in patients with bulky masses that precluded definitive direct endoscopic evaluation (12).

Three-dimensional reformations may also be used to display and calculate the volume of pharyngeal and laryngeal cancers. These data have proven useful in selecting treatment and evaluating tumor response to radiation and/or chemotherapy (13–15).

REFERENCES

1. Mukherji SK, Castillo M, Huda W, et al. Comparison of dynamic and spiral CT for imaging the glottic larynx. *J Comput Assist Tomogr* 1995;19(6):899–904.
2. Suojanen JN, Mukherji SK, Wippold FJ. Spiral CT of the larynx. *AJNR* 1994;15:1579–1582.
3. Craven CM, Naik KS, Blanshard KS, et al. Multispiral three-dimensional computed tomography in the investigation of craniosynostosis: technique optimization. *Br J Radiol* 1995;68:724–730.
4. Schmalfuss IM, Littwiler T, Mancuso AA. Fundamentals in head and neck imaging: CT protocols. In press.
5. Million RR, Cassissi. *Management of head and neck cancer: a multidisciplinary approach,* 2nd ed. Philadelphia: JB Lippincott, 1994;431–461.
6. Levy RA. Three-dimensional craniocervical helical CT: Is isotropic imaging possible? *Radiology* 1995;197: 645–648.
7. Spreer J, Krahe T, Jung G, et al. Spiral versus conventional CT in routine examinations of the neck. *J Comput Assist Tomogr* 1995;19(6):905–910.
8. Brink JA. Technical aspects of helical (spiral) CT. *Radiol Clin North Am* 1995;33(5):825–841.
9. Hermans R, Marchal G, Feenstra L, et al. Spiral CT of the temporal bone: value of image reconstruction at submillimetric table increments. *Neuroradiology* 1995;37:150–154.
10. Suojanen JN, Regan F. Spiral CT scanning of the paranasal sinuses. *AJNR* 1995;16:787–789.
11. Silverman PM, Zeiberg AS, Sessions RB, et al. Helical CT of the upper airway: normal and abnormal findings on three-dimensional reconstructed images. *AJR* 1995;165:541–546.
12. Silverman PM, Zeiberg AS, Sessions RB, Troost TR, Zeman RK. Three-dimensional (3-D) imaging of the hypopharynx and larynx using helical CT: comparison of radiological and otolaryngological evaluation. *Ann Otol Rhinol Otolaryngol* 1995;104(6):425–431.

13. Mukherji SK, Mancuso AA, Kotzur IK, et al. Radiologic appearance of the irradiated larynx. Part II. Primary site response. *Radiology* 1994;193:149–154.
14. Pameijer FA, Mancuso AA, Mendenhall WM, et al. Can pretreatment computed tomography predict local control in pyriform sinus carcinoma treated with definitive radiotherapy? *Head and Neck* 1998; In press.
15. Pameijer FA, Mancuso AA, Mendenhall WM, et al. Can pretreatment computed tomography predict local control in T3 squamous cell carcinoma of the glottic larynx treated with definitive radiotherapy? *Inter J Rad Onc and Biol* 1998; In press.

Protocol 1:
HEAD (Fig. 9)

INDICATION:	*Routine*
SCANNER SETTINGS:	kVp: 120 mAs: maximal; 240 if < 18 mos.
ORAL CONTRAST:	None
PHASE OF RESPIRATION:	Quiet breathing
SLICE THICKNESS:	5 mm in children; 7 mm in adults
PITCH:	1.0–1.4
HELICAL EXPOSURE TIME:	Depends on covered length
RECONSTRUCTION INTERVAL:	3 mm through the posterior fossa; 5 mm in children and 7 mm in adults through the rest of the head
SUPERIOR EXTENT:	Top of the head
INFERIOR EXTENT:	Foramen magnum

IV CONTRAST:

Concentration:	LOCM 300–320 mg iodine/mL or HOCM 282 mg iodine/mL (60% solution)
Rate:	0.5 mL/sec
Scan Delay:	5 min
Total Volume:	100 mL (adjust in children)

COMMENTS:

Note: No contrast used if hemorrhage, contusion, craniosynostosis, or hydrocephalus suspected.
DATA RECONSTRUCTION: Std.
SCOUT VIEW: Lateral
DISPLAY FOV: 21 cm in adults, 19 cm in children
SCAN FOV: Head
SCAN ANGLE: IOML
SAVE RAW DATA: Yes
Film in bone and soft-tissue windows.
DISPLAY FOV: 21 cm in adults, 19 cm in children
Consider three-dimensional reformations in patients with craniosynostosis. Change slice thickness to 1 mm and the gantry angle to 0 degrees for optimal quality of three-dimensional reformations.

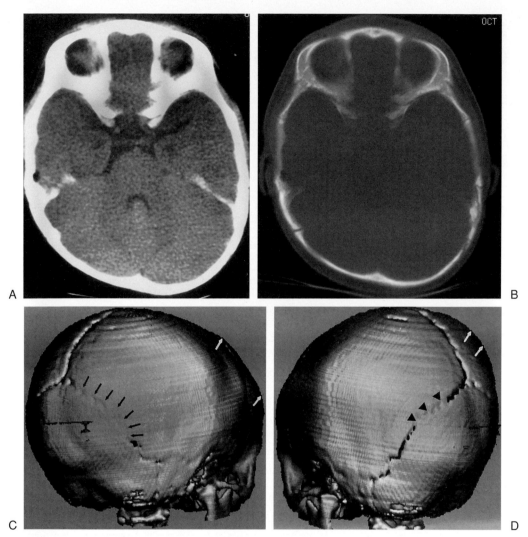

FIG. 9. Helical CT of a seven-month-old with malformed head was obtained with 3-mm slice thickness and a pitch of 1.4. The axial images filmed in soft tissue (**A**) and bone window (**B**) demonstrate the asymmetry of the skull in the occipital region. The three-dimensional images demonstrate the almost complete premature closure of the lambdoid suture on the right (*black arrows* in **C**) and lesser degrees of closure on the left (*arrowheads* in **D**). The slightly squared edges (*white arrows* in **C** and **D**) of each slice on the three-dimensional images (also known as the Lego effect) can be overcome by reconstructing the images with a smoothing algorithm or reduction of the slice thickness, preferably to 1 mm.

Protocol 2:
CAVERNOUS SINUS/SELLA

INDICATION:	*Suspected micro- or macroadenoma of the pituitary gland; mass in cavernous sinus, cavernous sinus thrombosis*
SCANNER SETTINGS:	kVp: 120 mAs: maximal
ORAL CONTRAST:	None
PHASE OF RESPIRATION:	Quiet breathing
SLICE THICKNESS:	3 mm through cavernous sinus in axial and coronal plane 7 mm through remainder of the head
PITCH:	1.0–1.4
HELICAL EXPOSURE TIME:	Depends on covered length
RECONSTRUCTION INTERVAL:	2 mm through cavernous sinus in axial and coronal plane 3 mm from hard palate to cavernous sinus 7 mm through remainder of the head

SUPERIOR EXTENT:	*Axial:*	*Coronal:*
INFERIOR EXTENT:	*Top of head* *Hard palate*	Posterior margin of globe IAC

IV CONTRAST:		
	Concentration:	LOCM 300–320 mg iodine/mL or HOCM 282 mg iodine/mL (60% solution)
	Rate:	1 mL/sec (45 mL bolus) 0.5 mL/sec (55 mL infusion)
	Scan Delay:	45 sec
	Total Volume:	100 mL

COMMENTS:

DATA RECONSTRUCTION: Std.
SCOUT VIEW: Lateral
DISPLAY FOV: 21 cm through entire head 10 cm through cavernous sinus in both planes
SCAN FOV: Head
SCAN ANGLE: *Axial:* IOML
                           Coronal: Perpendicular to IOML
SAVE RAW DATA: Yes, bone algorithm through cavernous sinus.
Film in bone and soft tissue windows.
Perform reformations of the axial images in coronal plane if patient is unable to tolerate direct coronal imaging.

Protocol 3:
TEMPORAL BONE (TB) WITHOUT IV CONTRAST (Fig. 10)

INDICATION: *Evaluation of trauma, congenital abnormalities, localized infectious or inflammatory disease; pulsatile tinnitus with visible middle ear mass on clinical examination; petrous apex mass*

SCANNER SETTINGS: kVp: 120
mAs: Maximal

ORAL CONTRAST: None

PHASE OF RESPIRATION: Quiet breathing

SLICE THICKNESS: 1 mm

PITCH: 1.0

HELICAL EXPOSURE TIME: Depends on covered length

RECONSTRUCTION INTERVAL: 0.5–1 mm

SUPERIOR EXTENT:
INFERIOR EXTENT:

Axial:	*Coronal:*
Top of TB	Anterior margin of TB
Hard palate	IAC
Tip of mastoid	Posterior margin of TB

IV CONTRAST: None

COMMENTS: **DATA RECONSTRUCTION:** Std.
SCOUT VIEW: Lateral
DISPLAY FOV: 9–10 cm
SCAN FOV: Head
SCAN ANGLE: *Axial:* IOML
Coronal: Perpendicular to IOML
SAVE RAW DATA: Yes, bone algorithm.
Film every image in bone and every third image in soft-tissue window.
Perform reformations of the axial images in coronal plane if patient is unable to tolerate direct coronal imaging.

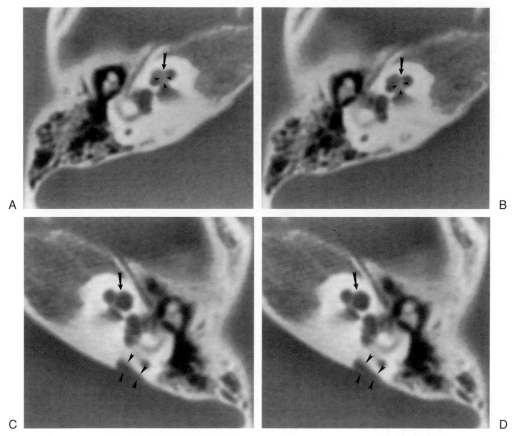

FIG. 10. Six-year-old child with left-sided hearing loss. The helical axial CT images were acquired with 1-mm slice thickness and a pitch of 1.0 and subsequently reconstructed as 0.5-mm contiguous sections. **A** and **B** demonstrate the excellent anatomic resolution of the normal right ear. The cochlea (*arrows* in **A** and **B**) is normally shaped with its two and one-half turns and contains a well-developed modiolus (*arrowheads* in **A** and **B**). **C** and **D** show the abnormal left ear, wherein the cochlear dysplasia (*arrows* in **C** and **D)** is manifest as deficient modiolus. Note the enlarged vestibular aqueduct (*arrowheads* in **C** and **D**).

Protocol 4:
TEMPORAL BONE (TB) WITH IV
CONTRAST

INDICATION: *Evaluation of infectious or inflammatory disease suspected to extend beyond the middle ear; pulsatile tinnitus without a visible middle ear mass on clinical examination; malignant tumor of the temporal bone*

SCANNER SETTINGS: kVp: 120
mAs: Maximal

ORAL CONTRAST: None

PHASE OF RESPIRATION: Quiet breathing

SLICE THICKNESS: 1 mm through temporal bone
5 mm through rest of the head and proximal neck

PITCH: 1.0

HELICAL EXPOSURE TIME: Depends on covered length

**RECONSTRUCTION
  INTERVAL:**   0.5–1 mm through temporal bone
3 mm through the upper and mid neck
5 mm to the top of the brain

SUPERIOR EXTENT:

INFERIOR EXTENT:

Axial:	*Coronal:*
Top of head	Orbital apex
Hard palate	IAC
C5 vertebral body	Occiput

IV CONTRAST:

Concentration:	LOCM 300–320 mg iodine/mL or HOCM 282 mg iodine/mL (60% solution)
Rate:	1 mL/sec (45 mL bolus) 0.5 mL/sec (105 mL infusion)
Scan Delay:	45 sec
Total Volume:	150 mL

COMMENTS:

DATA RECONSTRUCTION: Std.

SCOUT VIEW: Lateral

DISPLAY FOV: 9–10 cm through TB
                            19–21 cm through rest

SCAN FOV: Head

SCAN ANGLE: *Axial:* IOML
                          Coronal: Perpendicular to IOML

SAVE RAW DATA:

Yes, bone algorithm through TB. Film every image in bone and every third image in soft-tissue window through TB and all images in soft tissue through the rest.

Perform reformations of the axial images in coronal plane if patient is unable to tolerate direct coronal imaging.

Malignant tumors of TB:

Change superior extent to roof of the orbit and inferior extent to hard palate; obtain coronal images only through TB; include neck survey for evaluation of nodal disease.

Protocol 5:
ORBIT (Fig. 11)

INDICATION:	*Tumor, infection, orbital pathology*
SCANNER SETTINGS:	kVp: 120 mAs: Maximal
ORAL CONTRAST:	None
PHASE OF RESPIRATION:	Quiet breathing
SLICE THICKNESS:	3 mm
PITCH:	1.0
HELICAL EXPOSURE TIME:	Depends on covered length
RECONSTRUCTION INTERVAL:	1–3 mm

SUPERIOR EXTENT: ⎫
INFERIOR EXTENT: ⎭

Axial:	*Coronal:*
Top of frontal sinus	Ant. wall of frontal sinus
	Dorsum sellae
Hard palate	

IV CONTRAST:

Concentration:	LOCM 300–320 mg iodine/mL or HOCM 282 mg iodine/mL (60% solution)
Rate:	1 mL/sec (45 mL bolus) 0.5 mL/sec (55 mL infusion)
Scan Delay	45 sec
Total Volume	100 mL (adjust in children)

COMMENTS:

DATA RECONSTRUCTION: Std.
SCOUT VIEW: Lateral
DISPLAY FOV: 15–17 cm
SCAN FOV: Head
SCAN ANGLE: *Axial:* IOML
                  Coronal: Perpendicular to IOML
SAVE RAW DATA: Yes, bone algorithm.
Film in bone and soft-tissue windows.
Perform reformations of the axial images in coronal plane if patient is unable to tolerate direct coronal imaging.
Trauma or endocrine exophthalmus: No contrast.
Lesion limited to globe: Change superior extent to roof of the orbit and inferior extent to floor of the orbit; use 1 mm reconstruction interval; no imaging in coronal plane.
Retinoblastoma: Obtain images though the orbit without and with contrast using 1 mm reconstruction interval. Include imaging through the rest of the head. No imaging in coronal plane.
Varix suspected: Consider additional scanning with Valsalva maneuver or in prone position.

FIG. 11. Helical CT scan of a 5-year-old, cooperative child with clinical signs of cellulitis following repair of a deep laceration on the left face caused by a dog bite. The study was obtained to exclude postseptal infection or abscess. This helical CT scan was obtained in axial and direct coronal plane with 3-mm slice thickness and 1.0 pitch with intravenous contrast and without sedation. (**A**) The axial image demonstrates soft-tissue swelling over the left eye with stranding of the fatty tissue in the preseptal region (*). There are no signs of postseptal inflammation. The resolution of the brain and other soft tissue is good. (**B**) Direct coronal image through the mid-orbit is of excellent diagnostic quality without degradation by motion. (**C**) Reformatted image in the coronal plane without overlapping of the axial slices demonstrates markedly less anatomic detail than the direct coronal image. Additionally, some degradation is due to motion (*arrows*) that was present on two axial images used for this reformation. (**D**) The same coronal image as in **C** reformatted with 2-mm slice overlap exaggerates the motion artifacts (*arrows*). This is caused by additive effects of motion on the greater number of sections among those used for overlapped reformations.

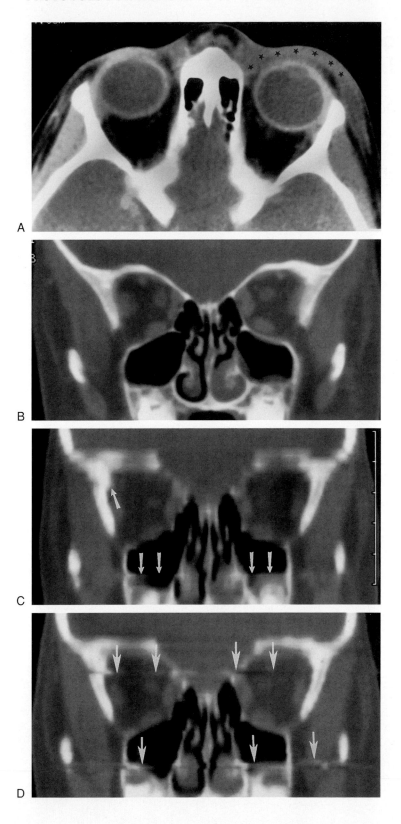

Protocol 6:
VISUAL PATHWAY

INDICATION:	*Suspected inflammatory disease, malignant or benign mass of the optic nerve, chiasm, visual tracts, and cortex*
SCANNER SETTINGS:	kVp: 120 mAs: Maximal
ORAL CONTRAST:	None
PHASE OF RESPIRATION:	Quiet breathing
SLICE THICKNESS:	3 mm through orbit; 5 mm through rest of head
PITCH:	1.0
HELICAL EXPOSURE TIME:	Depends on covered length
RECONSTRUCTION INTERVAL:	1 mm through orbit in axial plane 1 mm through the orbital apex and optic canal in coronal plane 3 mm through the anterior orbit in coronal plane 5 mm through remainder of head

SUPERIOR EXTENT:	*Axial:*	*Coronal:*
	Top of head	Posterior margin of globe
INFERIOR EXTENT:	Hard palate	Dorsum sellae

IV CONTRAST:		
	Concentration:	LOCM 300–320 mg iodine/mL or HOCM 282 mg iodine/mL (60% solution)
	Rate:	1 mL/sec (45 mL bolus) 0.5 mL/sec (55 mL infusion)
	Scan Delay:	45 sec
	Total Volume:	100 mL (adjust in children)

COMMENTS: **DATA RECONSTRUCTION:** Std.
SCOUT VIEW: Lateral
DISPLAY FOV: *Axial:* 15–17 cm through orbit
21 cm through head
Coronal: 15–17 cm
SCAN FOV: Head
SCAN ANGLE: *Axial:* IOML
Coronal: Perpendicular to IOML
SAVE RAW DATA: Yes, bone algorithm.
Film in bone and soft-tissue windows.
Perform reformations of the axial images in
coronal plane if patient is unable to tolerate
direct coronal imaging.

Protocol 7:
SINUSES/NASAL CAVITY WITHOUT IV CONTRAST (Fig. 12)

INDICATION:

Evaluation of routine infectious or inflammatory disease (e.g., patients with chronic sinusitis being considered for functional endoscopic sinus surgery)

SCANNER SETTINGS:

kVp: 120
mAs: 200

ORAL CONTRAST:

None

PHASE OF RESPIRATION:

Quiet breathing

SLICE THICKNESS:

3 mm

PITCH:

1.4

HELICAL EXPOSURE TIME:

Depends on covered length

RECONSTRUCTION INTERVAL:

3 mm

SUPERIOR EXTENT:
INFERIOR EXTENT:

Axial:	*Coronal:*
Top of frontal sinus	Ant. margin of frontal sinus
Bottom of maxilla	Dorsum sellae

IV CONTRAST:

None

COMMENTS:

DATA RECONSTRUCTION: Std.
SCOUT VIEW: Lateral
DISPLAY FOV: 15–17 cm
SCAN FOV: Head
SCAN ANGLE: *Axial:* IOML
                            Coronal: Perpendicular to IOML
SAVE RAW DATA: Yes, bone algorithm.
Film in bone and soft-tissue windows.
Perform reformations of the axial images in coronal plane if patient is unable to tolerate direct coronal imaging. Acquire the axial images with a pitch of 1.4 and slice thickness of 1 mm.

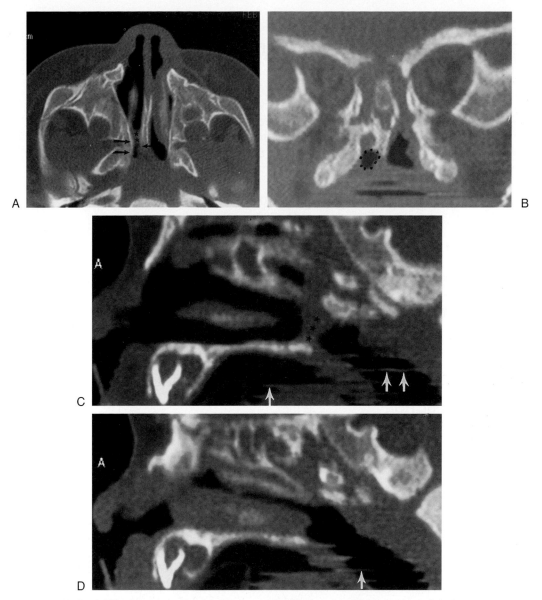

FIG. 12. Helical CT of a 2-month-old with nasal stuffiness was obtained in axial plane using a pitch of 1.0 and 1-mm slice thickness. Reformations in coronal and sagittal plane were obtained without slice overlap. (**A**) Axial image through the mid-nasal cavity shows bony narrowing of the choana (*arrows*) on the right with additional compromise of the nasal airway by a diaphragm of soft-tissue density (*). (**B**) The reformatted image in the coronal plane demonstrates the markedly reduced area of the nasal cavity on the right (*dotted line*) secondary to unilateral choanal atresia when compared with the left side. (**C,D**) Reformatted images in sagittal plane through the right (**C**) and left (**D**) nasal cavities confirm the soft-tissue obstruction of the right choana (*). Notice the marked linear artifacts (*arrows*) in the oral cavity and oropharynx that were caused by suction on a pacifier.

Protocol 8:
SINUSES/NASAL CAVITY WITH IV CONTRAST (Fig. 13)

INDICATION: *Evaluation of infectious or inflammatory disease suspected to extend beyond the sinuses to the brain or orbits; mucocele, benign or malignant tumor*

SCANNER SETTINGS: kVp: 120
mAs: 200

ORAL CONTRAST: None

PHASE OF RESPIRATION: Quiet breathing

SLICE THICKNESS: 3 mm

PITCH: 1.4

HELICAL EXPOSURE TIME: Depends on covered length

RECONSTRUCTION INTERVAL: 3 mm

SUPERIOR EXTENT:
INFERIOR EXTENT:

Axial:	*Coronal:*
Top of frontal sinus	Ant. margin of frontal sinus
Bottom of maxilla	Dorsum sellae

IV CONTRAST:

Concentration:	LOCM 300–320 mg iodine/mL or HOCM 282 mg iodine/mL (60% solution)
Rate:	1 mL/sec (45 mL bolus) 0.5 mL/sec (55 mL infusion)
Scan Delay:	45 sec
Total Volume:	100 mL

COMMENTS:

DATA RECONSTRUCTION: Std.
SCOUT VIEW: Lateral
DISPLAY FOV: 15–17 cm
SCAN FOV: Head
SCAN ANGLE: *Axial:* IOML
                      Coronal: Perpendicular to IOML
SAVE RAW DATA: Yes, bone algorithm.
Film in bone and soft-tissue windows.
Perform reformations of the axial images in coronal plane if patient is unable to tolerate direct coronal imaging. Acquire the axial images with a pitch of 1.4 and slice thickness of 1 mm.
Suspicion for sinus thrombosis: Include images through the rest of the head.
Malignant tumors: Include neck survey to evaluate for nodal disease.

FIG. 13. Helical CT of a 3-year-old with left-sided exophthalmus was obtained in axial and direct coronal plane (3-mm slice thickness, pitch of 1.0) with administration of intravenous contrast. The direct coronal images filmed in soft tissue (**A**) and bone (**B**) windows show a large mass (T) in the left nasal cavity. The tumor involves the ethmoid air cells on the left, infiltrates the left orbit (*large arrows*), and displaces the medial rectus muscle (*) laterally and the eye anteriorly. The tumor also extends to the superior aspect of the maxillary sinus (*arrowheads*), causing obstruction of the remaining portions (ms). Destruction of the left cribriform plate (*white arrow* in **B**) is also seen with tumor growth through this defect into the anterior cranial fossa (*small arrows*). (**C,D**) The reformatted images in coronal plane without slice overlap delineate the extent of the tumor into the orbit and sinuses; however, the growth into the anterior cranial fossa cannot be identified. The cribriform plate appears to be absent bilaterally (*arrows*). This mass was a biopsy-proven olfactory neuroblastoma.

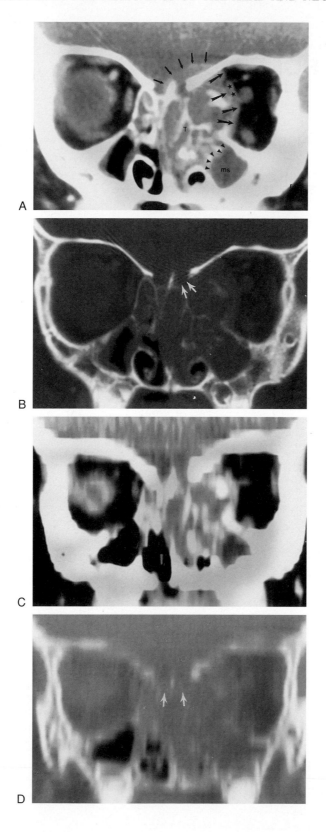

Protocol 9:
FACIAL BONES

INDICATION:	*Tumor, trauma, congenital*
SCANNER SETTINGS:	kVp: 120 mAs: 250
ORAL CONTRAST:	None
PHASE OF RESPIRATION:	Quiet breathing
SLICE THICKNESS:	3 mm
PITCH:	1.0
HELICAL EXPOSURE TIME:	Depends on covered length
RECONSTRUCTION INTERVAL:	3 mm

SUPERIOR EXTENT: ⎫
INFERIOR EXTENT: ⎬

Axial:	*Coronal:*
Top of frontal sinus	Ant. margin of frontal sinus
Bottom of mandible	Dorsum sellae

IV CONTRAST:	None
COMMENTS:	**DATA RECONSTRUCTION:** Std. **SCOUT VIEW:** Lateral **DISPLAY FOV:** 15–17 cm **SCAN FOV:** Head **SCAN ANGLE:** *Axial:* IOML *Coronal:* Perpendicular to IOML **SAVE RAW DATA:** Yes, bone algorithm. Film in bone and soft-tissue windows. Perform reformations of the axial images in coronal plane if patient is unable to tolerate direct coronal imaging. Acquire the axial images with a pitch of 1.4 and slice thickness of 1 mm.

Protocol 10: NASOPHARYNX/PARAPHARYNGEAL SPACE/ MASTICATOR SPACE

INDICATION:	*Tumor, inflammatory disease, infection*
SCANNER SETTINGS:	kVp: 120 mAs: Maximal
ORAL CONTRAST:	None
PHASE OF RESPIRATION:	Quiet breathing
SLICE THICKNESS:	3 mm
PITCH:	1.0
HELICAL EXPOSURE TIME:	Depends on covered length
RECONSTRUCTION INTERVAL:	3 mm

	Axial:	*Coronal:*
SUPERIOR EXTENT:	Top of sella	Middle of hard palate
INFERIOR EXTENT:	Hyoid bone	Posterior margin of clivus

IV CONTRAST:

Concentration:	LOCM 300–320 mg iodine/mL or HOCM 282 mg iodine/mL (60% solution)
Rate:	1 mL/sec (45 mL bolus) 0.5 mL/sec (105 mL infusion)
Scan Delay:	45 sec
Total Volume:	150 mL

COMMENTS:

DATA RECONSTRUCTION: Std.

SCOUT VIEW: Lateral

DISPLAY FOV: 16–19 cm

SCAN FOV: Head

SCAN ANGLE: *Axial:* IOML and parallel to the long axis of the mandible (change angle around teeth)
Coronal: Perpendicular to IOML

SAVE RAW DATA: Yes, bone algorithm through skull base. Film all images in soft-tissue window and only the images through the skull base in bone window.

Perform reformations of the axial images through the skull base in coronal plane if patient is unable to tolerate direct coronal imaging. Acquire the axial images with a pitch of 1.4 and slice thickness of 1 mm.

Infectious or inflammatory disease: No coronal images. Continue scanning through the upper chest if retropharyngeal abscess present.

Malignant tumors: Include neck survey to evaluate for nodal disease.

Reconstruct in 1–2-mm intervals through the skull base in patients with nasopharyngeal cancer and suspicion for central skull base involvement.

Protocol 11:
PAROTID GLAND

INDICATION:	*Tumor, inflammatory disease, infection*
SCANNER SETTINGS:	kVp: 120 mAs: Maximal
ORAL CONTRAST:	None
PHASE OF RESPIRATION:	Quiet breathing
SLICE THICKNESS:	3 mm
PITCH:	1.0
HELICAL EXPOSURE TIME:	Depends on covered length
RECONSTRUCTION INTERVAL:	3 mm
SUPERIOR EXTENT:	Bottom of the sella
INFERIOR EXTENT:	Hyoid bone

IV CONTRAST:

Concentration:	LOCM 300–320 mg iodine/mL or HOCM 282 mg iodine/mL (60% solution)
Rate:	1 mL/sec (45-mL bolus) 0.5 mL/sec (105-mL infusion)
Scan Delay:	45 sec
Total Volume:	150 mL

COMMENTS:

DATA RECONSTRUCTION: Std.

SCOUT VIEW: Lateral

DISPLAY FOV: 16–19 cm

SCAN FOV: Head

SCAN ANGLE: IOML and parallel to the long axis of the mandible (change angle around teeth)

SAVE RAW DATA: Yes, bone algorithm through skull base. Film all images in soft-tissue window and only the images through the skull base in bone window.

Malignant tumors: Include neck survey to evaluate for nodal disease.

With facial nerve palsy: Include scanning through temporal bone (see specific protocol) and reconstruct in 1-mm intervals through the parotid gland.

Protocol 12:
SOFT/HARD PALATE

INDICATION: *Tumor, inflammatory disease, infection*

SCANNER SETTINGS: kVp: 120
                               mAs: Maximal

ORAL CONTRAST: None

PHASE OF RESPIRATION: Quiet breathing

SLICE THICKNESS: 3 mm

PITCH: 1.0

HELICAL EXPOSURE TIME: Depends on covered length

**RECONSTRUCTION
   INTERVAL:**   3 mm

SUPERIOR EXTENT: ⎫   *Axial:*   *Coronal:*
                     ⎬   Bottom of the   Ant. margin of hard palate
INFERIOR EXTENT: ⎭   sella   Dorsum sellae
                               Hyoid bone

IV CONTRAST:

Concentration:	LOCM 300–320 mg iodine/mL or HOCM 282 mg iodine/mL (60% solution)
Rate:	1 mL/sec (45 mL bolus) 0.5 mL/sec (105 mL infusion)
Scan Delay:	45 sec
Total Volume:	150 mL

COMMENTS:

DATA RECONSTRUCTION: Std.
SCOUT VIEW: Lateral
DISPLAY FOV: 16–19 cm
SCAN FOV: Head
SCAN ANGLE: *Axial:* IOML and parallel to the long axis of the mandible (change angle around teeth)
Coronal: Perpendicular to IOML
SAVE RAW DATA: Yes, bone algorithm through hard palate. Film all images in soft-tissue window and only the images through the hard palate in bone window.

Perform reformations of the axial images through the hard palate in coronal plane if patient is unable to tolerate direct coronal imaging. Acquire the axial images with a pitch of 1.4 and slice thickness of 1 mm.

Malignant tumors: Include neck survey to evaluate for nodal disease.

Protocol 13:
OROPHARYNX/ORAL CAVITY/FLOOR OF THE MOUTH (Fig. 14)

INDICATION:	*Excluding soft and hard palate*
SCANNER SETTINGS:	kVp: 120 mAs: Maximal
ORAL CONTRAST:	None
PHASE OF RESPIRATION:	Quiet breathing
SLICE THICKNESS:	3 mm
PITCH:	1.0
HELICAL EXPOSURE TIME:	Depends on covered length
RECONSTRUCTION INTERVAL:	3 mm
SUPERIOR EXTENT:	Floor of the orbit
INFERIOR EXTENT:	Hyoid bone

IV CONTRAST:		
	Concentration:	LOCM 300–320 mg iodine/mL or HOCM 282 mg iodine/mL (60% solution)
	Rate:	1 mL/sec (45 mL bolus) 0.5 mL/sec (105 mL infusion)
	Scan Delay:	45 sec
	Total Volume:	150 mL

COMMENTS:

DATA RECONSTRUCTION: Std.
SCOUT VIEW: Lateral
DISPLAY FOV: 16–19 cm
SCAN FOV: Head
SCAN ANGLE: IOML and parallel to the long axis of the mandible (change angle around teeth)
SAVE RAW DATA: Yes, bone algorithm through mandible. Film all images in soft-tissue window

and only the images through the mandible in bone window.

Infectious or inflammatory disease in the floor of the mouth: Obtain also coronal images with a pitch of 1.0 and slice thickness of 3 mm through the oral cavity.

Malignant tumors: Include neck survey to evaluate for nodal disease.

Obtain 1–2 mm reconstruction interval through the mandible in patients with oral cavity tumors and suspicion for mandibular involvement.

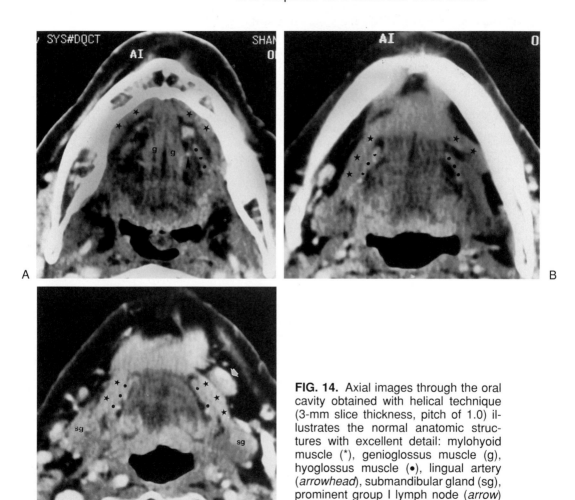

FIG. 14. Axial images through the oral cavity obtained with helical technique (3-mm slice thickness, pitch of 1.0) illustrates the normal anatomic structures with excellent detail: mylohyoid muscle (*), genioglossus muscle (g), hyoglossus muscle (•), lingual artery (*arrowhead*), submandibular gland (sg), prominent group I lymph node (*arrow*) on the left.

Protocol 14:
MANDIBLE

INDICATION:	*Trauma, infection, and tumor*
SCANNER SETTINGS:	kVp: 120 mAs: 250
ORAL CONTRAST:	None
PHASE OF RESPIRATION:	Quiet breathing
SLICE THICKNESS:	1 mm
PITCH:	1.4
HELICAL EXPOSURE TIME:	Depends on covered length
RECONSTRUCTION INTERVAL:	1 mm
SUPERIOR EXTENT:	Temporomandibular Joint
INFERIOR EXTENT:	Inferior margin of the mandible

IV CONTRAST:

Concentration:	LOCM 300–320 mg iodine/mL or HOCM 282 mg iodine/mL (60% solution)
Rate:	1 mL/sec (45 mL bolus) 0.5 mL/sec (55 mL infusion)
Scan Delay:	45 sec
Total Volume:	100 mL

COMMENTS:

DATA RECONSTRUCTION: Std.
SCOUT VIEW: Lateral
DISPLAY FOV: 16–18 cm
SCAN FOV: Head
SCAN ANGLE: IOML
SAVE RAW DATA: Yes, bone algorithm.
Film every image in bone and every third image
in soft-tissue window.
Consider dental reformations of the mandible.

Protocol 15:
HYPOPHARYNX/LARYNX (Fig. 15)

INDICATION:	*Tumor, trauma, and infection*
SCANNER SETTINGS:	kVp: 120 mAs: 280–300
ORAL CONTRAST:	None
PHASE OF RESPIRATION:	Quiet breathing
SLICE THICKNESS:	3 mm
PITCH:	1.4
HELICAL EXPOSURE TIME:	Depends on covered length
RECONSTRUCTION INTERVAL:	3 mm
SUPERIOR EXTENT:	Midportion of the mandible body
INFERIOR EXTENT:	Lung apex

IV CONTRAST:

Concentration:	LOCM 300–320 mg iodine/mL or HOCM 282 mg iodine/mL (60% solution)
Rate:	1 mL/sec (45 mL bolus) 0.5 mL/sec (105 mL infusion)
Scan Delay:	45 sec
Total Volume:	150 mL

COMMENTS:

DATA RECONSTRUCTION: Std.
SCOUT VIEW: Lateral
DISPLAY FOV: 10 cm through the larynx, 16–19 cm through the entire scanned area
SCAN FOV: Head
SCAN ANGLE: Parallel to the long axis of the true vocal cords. If these can not be identified, scan parallel to the C4/5 or C5/6 disc space.
SAVE RAW DATA: Yes, bone algorithm through the larynx. Film all images in soft-tissue

window and only the images through the larynx in bone window.

Trauma/subglottic stenosis: No contrast. Consider reformations in coronal and sagittal plane or in three dimensions.

Malignant tumors: Consider three-dimensional reformations to better determine the relation to adjacent anatomic structures and tumor volume.

Perform 1–2-mm thin sections from the false vocal cord to the bottom of the cricoid cartilage in patients with small-volume tumors or questionable extent of the tumor into the laryngeal ventricle and/or subglottic region.

Consider coronal reformations at 1–2-mm intervals in patients with vocal cord cancer.

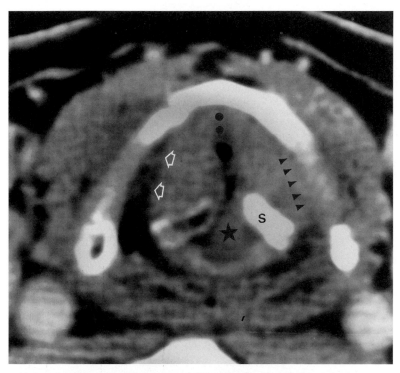

FIG. 15. Axial CT image obtained with helical technique (3-mm slice thickness, pitch of 1.0) shows the true vocal cords in closed position. The paraglottic fat plane on the left is completely obliterated (*arrowheads*) by an infiltrating tumor in the left true vocal cord. The normal paraglottic fat is clearly visualized on the right (*white arrows*). Occasionally, the obliterated paraglottic fat plane might be the only sign of an abnormality in this region. In this patient, however, there is also significant sclerosis of the left arytenoid cartilage (s), which might be reactive or due to tumor invasion. The anterior (•) and posterior (*) commissures appear very thickened on this image, suggesting that the tumor is extending to the right side. However, the thickness of the commissures should never be evaluated with the true vocal cords in closed position.

Protocol 16:
NECK SURVEY (Fig. 16)

INDICATION:	*Neck mass of unknown etiology, lymph node survey, lymphoma, unknown primary, skin cancer, melanoma*
SCANNER SETTINGS:	kVp: 120 mAs: Maximal
ORAL CONTRAST:	None
PHASE OF RESPIRATION:	Quiet breathing
SLICE THICKNESS:	3 mm
PITCH:	1.4
HELICAL EXPOSURE TIME:	Depends on covered length
RECONSTRUCTION INTERVAL:	3 mm
SUPERIOR EXTENT:	Top of sella
INFERIOR EXTENT:	Lung apex

IV CONTRAST:

Concentration:	LOCM 300–320 mg iodine/mL or HOCM 282 mg iodine/mL (60% solution)
Rate:	1 mL/sec (45 mL bolus) 0.5 mL/sec (105 mL infusion)
Scan Delay:	45 sec
Total Volume:	150 mL

COMMENTS:

DATA RECONSTRUCTION: Std.
SCOUT VIEW: Lateral
DISPLAY FOV: 16–19 cm
SCAN FOV: Head
SCAN ANGLE: IOML and parallel to the long axis of the mandible (change angle around teeth)
SAVE RAW DATA: Yes. Film all images in soft-tissue window.
Skin cancer/melanoma: DFOV should include the posterior neck on each slice.

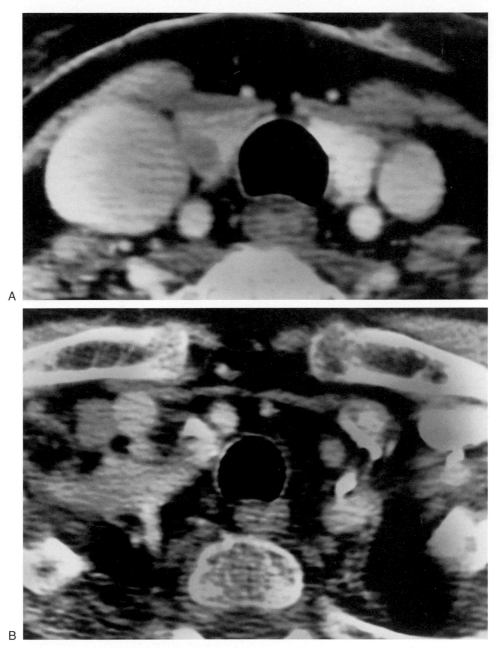

FIG. 16. Axial CT images performed with helical technique (3-mm slice thickness, pitch of 1.0) in a patient with small body habitus demonstrate acceptable anatomic detail in the lower neck (**A**) and at the thoracic inlet (**B**). This region is often degraded by artifacts caused by the shoulders of patients with average or large body habitus and/or short necks. Scanning of this region with conventional technique, with twice the usual mAs, is frequently required for optimal image quality. Incidental low-attenuation area is seen in right thyroid lobe.

Protocol 17:
SUSPECTED CSF LEAK (Fig. 17)

INDICATION:	*CSF otorrhea and/or rhinorrhea*
SCANNER SETTINGS:	kVp: 120
	mAs: 300-maximal
ORAL CONTRAST:	None
PHASE OF RESPIRATION:	Quiet breathing
SLICE THICKNESS:	1 mm
PITCH:	1.4
HELICAL EXPOSURE TIME:	Depends on covered length
RECONSTRUCTION **INTERVAL:**	1 mm

SUPERIOR EXTENT: ⎫
⎬
INFERIOR EXTENT: ⎭
	Axial:
	Top of frontal
	   sinus
	Hard palate
		Coronal:
		Ant. margin of frontal sinus
		Posterior margin of mastoid
		   air cells

IV CONTRAST:	None
COMMENTS:	**DATA RECONSTRUCTION:** Std.

SCOUT VIEW: Lateral
DISPLAY FOV: 15–17 cm for CSF rhinorrhea
                        9–10 cm for CSF otorrhea
SCAN FOV: Head
SCAN ANGLE: *Axial:* IOML
                        Coronal: Perpendicular to IOML
SAVE RAW DATA: Yes, bone algorithm.
Film every image in bone and every third image
   in soft-tissue windows.
Perform reformations of the axial images in
   coronal plane if patient is unable to tolerate
   direct coronal imaging.
Consider intrathecal contrast.
CSF rhinorrhea: Change the inferior extent of
   scanning in axial plane to mid orbit and the
   posterior extent of imaging in coronal to
   dorsum sellae.
CSF otorrhea: Change the superior extent of
   scanning in axial plane to top of sella and the
   anterior extent of imaging in coronal to anterior
   margin of the temporal bone.

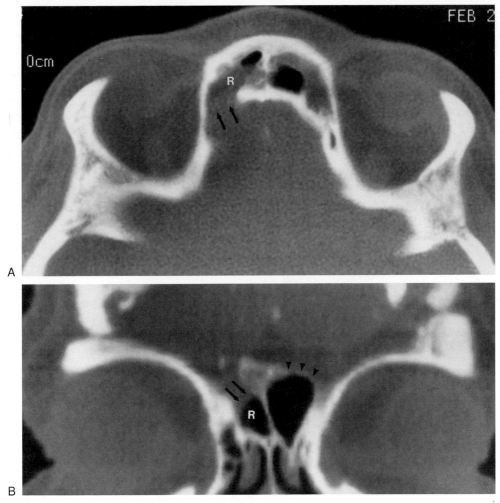

FIG. 17. Helical CT scan in a patient with rhinorrhea and inability to tolerate direct coronal imaging. The axial images (**A**) were obtained with 1-mm slice thickness and a pitch of 1.4. The coronal reformations (**B**) were performed without slice overlap. Both images demonstrate a large defect (*arrows*) in the postero-superior aspect of the right frontal sinus (R), the site of the CSF leak. The roof of the left frontal sinus (*arrowheads*) can be seen as intact on this reformatted image.

Protocol 18:
CERVICAL SPINE: CT MYELOGRAM

INDICATION:	*Neck pain, disk disease, infection, trauma, degenerative disease*
SCANNER SETTINGS:	kVp: 120 mAs: 250
ORAL CONTRAST:	None
PHASE OF RESPIRATION:	Quiet breathing
SLICE THICKNESS:	3 mm
PITCH:	1.0
HELICAL EXPOSURE TIME:	Depends on covered length
RECONSTRUCTION INTERVAL:	3 mm
SUPERIOR EXTENT:	One disc space above the level of radiculopathy determined on clinical examination and/or myelography
INFERIOR EXTENT:	One disc space below the level of radiculopathy determined on clinical examination and/or myelography
IV CONTRAST:	None
COMMENTS:	**DATA RECONSTRUCTION:** Std. **SCOUT VIEW:** Lateral **DISPLAY FOV:** 21 cm in adults, 19 cm in children **SCAN FOV:** Head **SCAN ANGLE:** None **SAVE RAW DATA:** Yes, bone algorithm. Film in bone and soft-tissue windows. Perform reformations along the plane of disc spaces. Consider reformations in coronal and sagittal plane. Abnormalities of C1 and 2: Consider scanning with 1-mm slice thickness and a pitch of 1.4.

Protocol 19:
EXTRACRANIAL VASCULATURE

INDICATION:	*Vascular stenosis, aneurysm, malformation, and trauma*
SCANNER SETTINGS:	kVp: 120 mAs: 250
ORAL CONTRAST:	None
PHASE OF RESPIRATION:	Quiet breathing
SLICE THICKNESS:	1 mm
PITCH:	1.5
HELICAL EXPOSURE TIME:	Depends on covered length
RECONSTRUCTION INTERVAL:	1 mm
SUPERIOR EXTENT:	Skull base
INFERIOR EXTENT:	C6 vertebral body

IV CONTRAST:

Concentration:	LOCM 300–320 mg iodine/mL or HOCM 282 mg iodine/mL (60% solution)
Rate:	3 mL/sec
Scan Delay:	20 sec
Total Volume:	150 mL

COMMENTS:

DATA RECONSTRUCTION: Soft tissue
SCOUT VIEW: Lateral
DISPLAY FOV: 15 cm
SCAN FOV: Head
SCAN ANGLE: None
SAVE RAW DATA: Yes.
Perform data processing using maximum-intensity projection (MIP) technique and display the data in three dimensions and various angles.

Protocol 20:
INTRACRANIAL VASCULATURE (Circle of Willis) (Fig. 18)

INDICATION:	*Aneurysm, stenosis, vascular malformation*
SCANNER SETTINGS:	kVp: 120 mAs: 250
ORAL CONTRAST:	None
PHASE OF RESPIRATION:	Quiet breathing
SLICE THICKNESS:	1 mm
PITCH:	1.0
HELICAL EXPOSURE TIME:	Depends on covered length
RECONSTRUCTION INTERVAL:	1 mm
SUPERIOR EXTENT:	Top of third ventricle
INFERIOR EXTENT:	Skull base

IV CONTRAST:

Concentration:	LOCM 300–320 mg iodine/mL or HOCM 282 mg iodine/mL (60% solution)
Rate:	3 mL/sec
Scan Delay:	20 sec for arteries
Total Volume:	100 mL

COMMENTS:

DATA RECONSTRUCTION: Soft tissue
SCOUT VIEW: Lateral
DISPLAY FOV: 15 cm
SCAN FOV: Head
SCAN ANGLE: None
SAVE RAW DATA: Yes.
Perform data processing using maximum-intensity projection (MIP) technique and display the data in three dimensions and various angles.

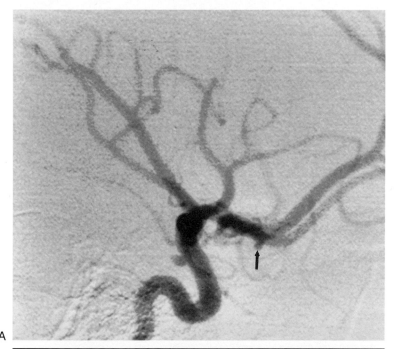

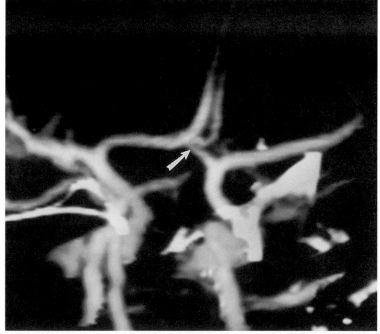

FIG. 18. (**A**) This patient presented with subarachnoid hemorrhage due to an arteriovenous malformation (AVM). The angiogram demonstrated the AVM (not shown) and a questionable small anterior communicating artery aneurysm (*black arrow*), which was visualized in multiple but not all different projections. (**B**) An angio-CT of the circle of Willis was done for confirmation using helical technique using the preceding protocol. The three-dimensional reformations could not reveal an aneurysm but did show a tortuous left ACA (*white arrow*) that most likely mimicked an aneurysm on the angiogram.

Helical (Spiral) Computed Tomography,
edited by Paul M. Silverman.
Lippincott–Raven Publishers, Philadelphia © 1998.

3

Protocols for Helical CT of the Chest

Philip Costello* and David P. Naidich**

*Department of Radiology, The Queen Elizabeth Hospital, Adelaide,
South Australia 5011
**Department of Radiology, Bellevue Hospital, New York, New York 10016

Helical computed tomography (CT) was introduced into clinical practice in 1990, with the chest being the first area investigated (1). Subsequent evaluation has more than justified initial enthusiasm. Primarily the result of improved temporal resolution due to acquisition of data in a single breath-hold (resulting in reduced misregistration and respiratory and cardiac motion artifacts and elimination of variation in the depth of respiration between scans) and longitudinal (z-axis) resolution due to the ability to acquire overlapping reconstructions, helical scanning has indeed transformed our ability to evaluate chest disease (2–4).

It is also apparent that widespread availability of helical CT has led to considerable uncertainty about optimal utilization both for routine CT examinations and for more specialized applications. This is because the ability to acquire data volumetrically means that a nearly limitless variety of potential scan protocols is now available for axial imaging (5). Variables that need to be selected include collimation, pitch, breath-hold period, field of view, reconstruction interval (or index), rate and volume of intravenous contrast administration, reconstruction algorithm, and radiation dose. It is axiomatic that no single set of optimal scan parameters is sufficient for all CT applications (6). Rather, a variety of protocols exist that have been individually tailored to specific clinical indications. Although many of these reflect personal or institutional preferences, a few basic principles usually apply.

First, it is generally preferable to obtain thinner sections using a larger pitch than to take thicker sections with a smaller pitch. As will be discussed, this is especially applicable to studies in which the main indication is assessment of potentially occult disease involving small anatomic structures, such as the airways or lung parenchyma. Second, as a general rule, optimal longitudinal (z-axis) resolution for lesion detection requires that at least two images be reconstructed per 360 degrees of tube rotation. This feature is unique to helical CT and, as will be discussed, has led to the development of numerous retrospective reconstruction techniques of real and potential clinical value that were not possible or practical with conventional CT (CCT). For example, three-dimensional data sets are now routinely reconstructed, and CT angiography is commonly used as an alternative to intra-arterial digital subtraction angiography for investigation of vascular disease.

For purposes of organization, the following discussion will focus first on vascular applications, particularly the use of helical CT to diagnose pulmonary emboli and aortic disease. Following this, attention will be directed to the variety of protocols needed for optimal evaluation of airway disease, both central and peripheral. Finally, current concepts in helical CT applications to focal lung disease will be discussed, as will optimal methods for performing high-resolution CT in patients with diffuse infiltrative lung disease (DILD).

VASCULAR DISEASE

Intravenous Contrast Administration

Many clinical indications for thoracic CT require the intravenous injection of iodinated contrast material. The purpose of contrast is to differentiate normal vascular mediastinal and hilar structures from pathological conditions. Lung cancer staging, detection of lymphadenopathy, and differentiation of normal vascular structures such as pulmonary arteries from lymph nodes all require intravenous contrast administration. Many patients referred for oncological assessment have concurrent examinations involving the neck and liver, both of which require contrast enhancement for detection of pathological conditions. Since helical CT acquisition times are at least four times as fast as conventional CT, new strategies to optimize contrast material have been developed.

A complete helical CT thoracic examination can be performed with as little as 60 mL of 300 mg I/mL (7). A recent study showed that reduced iodine concentration actually improved arterial enhancement (8). Rubin and colleagues showed that 100 mL of 150-mg I/mL contrast material achieved by diluting a 50-mL vial of 300-mg I/mL concentration with 50 mL normal saline resulted in scans of superior quality compared with the same undiluted dose (300 mg I/mL) (8). A greater degree of mediastinal arterial enhancement and reduction in perivenous artifacts led to better-quality thoracic CT scans with 150 mg I/mL concentration. Schneider has also found that using a flow rate of 3 mL/sec with 150 mg I/mL provides images of high quality with excellent opacification of the ascending and descending aortas and pulmonary arteries (9). A dilute contrast material protocol is employed in studies limited to the thorax alone and for the detection of pulmonary emboli. Departments using nonionic contrast material exclusively will realize significant cost savings with the 150 mg/mL iodine concentration protocol. A larger number of thoracic studies are performed in conjunction with examinations of the neck, abdomen, and pelvis, where 300 mg I/mL concentration is needed.

In most instances a 12–18-sec scan delay provides excellent opacification of the pulmonary arteries and aorta. Because optimal scan delay will vary, however, in patients with questionably abnormal cardiac output, a test injection may be obtained using regions of interest to determine peak vessel enhancement. In our experience this is best accomplished with a test dose of 20 mL with images obtained every 5 sec for a total of 25 sec when evaluating the pulmonary arteries, and every 10 sec for a total of 40 sec when evaluating the aorta.

New hardware and software (e.g., computer automated scanning technology as reported by Silverman and colleagues) have been incorporated into CT scanners that allow the user to monitor vascular enhancement during the injection of contrast material (10). This approach provides the most efficient use of contrast without requiring a test dose. The technique employs low-dose scans obtained with a rapid reconstruction interval, so that Hounsfield unit (HU) measurements can be made quickly, establishing a desired threshold of enhancement and providing timing of mediastinal vessel enhancement despite a variable cardiac output. Contrast should always be injected through a 20-gauge or 21-gauge angiocath system via a basilic vein providing the most direct communication with the axillary and subclavian veins. Prior to connecting to an extension tubing, a bolus injection of 5–10 mL of sterile saline may be of value to detect possible extravasation.

PULMONARY EMBOLISM

Much enthusiasm for helical CT in the detection of pulmonary embolism was generated by the first study of 42 patients, which compared helical CT to pulmonary angiography (11).

The overall sensitivity and specificity for helical CT in detecting central pulmonary emboli were 100% and 96%, respectively, but this first study excluded branches obscured by partial volume averaging. A recent, larger prospective study of 75 patients reported a sensitivity of 91% and a specificity of 78% (12). This later study did not exclude patients with partial volume-averaging problems, and technical failures observed in 10 patients accounted for a lower sensitivity. Helical CT can definitively show emboli to the level of segmental vessels, and the CT signs of acute emboli are based on a modification of Sinner's description (13). Partial filling defects are central or marginal areas of low attenuation surrounded by contrast material. Complete filling defects are defined as intraluminal areas of low attenuation not surrounded by contrast material. Mural defects are defined as peripheral areas of low attenuation, and the railway track sign defines a freely floating clot in the vessel lumen. The main advantage of helical CT over conventional angiography is that it permits direct visualization of a thrombus in a transverse plane.

To interpret helical CT images accurately, a comprehensive understanding of bronchovascular segmental anatomy is important, as is the usual size and location of hilar lymph nodes, which may mimic emboli (14). Obliquely oriented vessels particularly in the middle lobe and lingula can lead to difficulties in detecting emboli, but multiplanar reformations may help (15). Multiplanar reformations of obliquely oriented vessels allow for imaging the lung in a longitudinal axis and help differentiate a filling defect due to intraluminal thrombus from extrinsic hilar masses.

Helical CT is a fast, noninvasive way to diagnose acute thromboemboli by avoiding the risks associated with angiography, which include cardiac arrhythmias, perforation, and rarely, death. Patients known to be at high risk for the complications of pulmonary angiography and those who are seriously ill are likely to benefit from the use of helical CT. Patients with clinical evidence of massive emboli can be screened by contrast-enhanced helical CT. Although 9% of CT scans can be inconclusive for the diagnosis of emboli, insufficient visualization of pulmonary arteries has been reported in as many as 12% of completed angiograms, the so-called gold standard (16). A major limitation of helical CT is the diagnosis of subsegmental emboli that are beyond the limit of transverse CT imaging. However, isolated peripheral subsegmental clots appear to be an infrequent clinical situation, occurring in only 5% of patients studied by Rémy-Jardin (12). Patients without a history of prior cardiac or pulmonary disease are felt not to have a high morbidity risk for isolated subsegmental emboli, and the need for treating such individuals is controversial.

Further clarification of the role of helical CT compared with ventilation perfusion (V-P) scanning as a noninvasive screening procedure is needed. Rémy-Jardin found that one of 25 patients studied had a normal ventilation perfusion scan but that a large central clot was revealed by helical CT and angiography (12). Data from electron beam CT and V-P scans and pulmonary angiography have shown the sensitivity and specificity of CT to be 65% and 97% compared with V-P scan sensitivity of 20% and specificity 52% (17). A noninvasive procedure with a greater sensitivity and specificity than ventilation perfusion scans is required to diagnose pulmonary embolism. Further larger studies are needed to confirm the high sensitivity and accuracy of fast scanning techniques for the diagnosis of thromboembolic disease. These techniques will probably replace V-P lung scanning as the initial screening test.

Patients with chronic thromboembolic hypertension can be diagnosed on helical CT, and CT can be used as a complement to pulmonary angiography prior to surgical intervention (18,19). Pulmonary angiography can miss mural thrombi caused by regular concentric narrowing of the arterial lumen. Helical CT is not, however, as accurate as angiography in the analysis of the peripheral arterial bed, but central vascular abnormalities secondary to organized thrombi are well shown. In addition to the vascular changes of chronic embolism, attenuation changes in the lung parenchyma may be observed. Regional hyperattenuation areas in the lung parenchyma have been shown to correlate with dilated feeding segmental arteries representing hyperperfused lung in chronic embolism (18).

AORTIC DISEASE

Aortic Dissection

Precise definition of the site of a tear and extent of involvement are principal determinants of the patient's course, prognosis, and treatment. Precontrast sections are obtained, to detect both displacement of intimal calcification and high attenuation aortic wall containing fresh hemorrhage. Helical CT has many advantages when imaging patients are suspected of aortic dissection (3,20). Arterial phase imaging makes the intimal flaps, entry points, aortic cobwebs, and branch vessel involvement easier to identify (21). Reconstruction of overlapping images provides multiplanar sections, which can make entry points more conspicuous through partial volume elimination. Multiplanar images are done first because it is much easier to depict the relationship of intimal flaps to aortic branch vessels than to try to show the relationship using transverse sections alone (3,20,22). Curved planar reformations are also reconstructed to show the intimal flap, false channel, and hematoma extension better than catheter angiography. Quint and colleagues found helical CT with multiplanar reformations valuable in predicting which patients would need hypothermic circulatory arrest, particularly when there is involvement of the aortic arch (22). Radiologists should be aware of a unique artifact in the ascending aorta that can mimic aortic dissection (23). It results from expansion contraction of the ascending aorta and is seen more with heart rates averaging between 0.6 and 1.0/sec.

In most patients, helical CT can replace angiography for the diagnosis of aortic dissection (3,20,24,25). Angiography can demonstrate coronary artery involvement and aortic valve competency, but branch vessel involvement can be demonstrated on multiplanar CT and three-dimensional images.

Both magnetic resonance imaging (MRI) and transesophageal echocardiography (TEE) are highly accurate alternative diagnostic options (26). Patient motion, irregular respirations, or poor ECG gating may limit MRI image quality, and many life support and monitoring devices essential to these patients cannot be brought into an MRI suite. These problems limit MRI's role for many acutely ill patients suspected of aortic dissection. Although transesophageal echocardiography combined with transthoracic echocardiography has a high sensitivity and specificity for dissection, not all departments have personnel 24 hours a day who have the expertise to do this procedure. An important potential limitation of TEE is the presence of a relatively blind zone involving a portion of the ascending aorta due to obscuration by air within the adjacent trachea. Ultimately, the final choice of an imaging modality for aortic dissection depends upon the speed and reliability with which studies can be performed and interpreted in a specific clinical environment (26). In most institutions, helical CT is the imaging modality of choice for an acutely ill patient.

Aortic Aneurysms

Thoracic aortic aneurysms, particularly those arising adjacent to the great vessels or the infralateral aspect of the arch, need to be clearly defined to determine which type of surgical procedure should be performed. Helical CT with multiplanar and three-dimensional reformations allows the relationship between aortic aneurysms and branch vessels to be clearly defined

(3,24,27). Reconstruction of overlapping sections reduces the volume-averaging phenomenon of thick-slice conventional CT and allows clear definition of calcification, thrombus, and contrast material.

CT angiography may play a valuable role following stent placement and graft procedures. Periaortic leaks around graft anastomoses or stents can be delineated by the demonstration of extravasation of contrast material. Catheter angiography is less valuable than helical CT, because these areas of extravasation tend to be slow-flow leaks. CT may also be of value in cases with suspected penetrating atheromatous ulcers (28).

AIRWAY DISEASE/HILAR EVALUATION TECHNIQUES

Scan Acquisition

In our experience it is helpful to visualize the chest as divided into three zones whenever the airways are the principal focus of the CT examination. These include (a) an apical zone (extending from the thoracic inlet to just above the carina); (b) a hilar zone (extending from just above the carina to the level of the inferior pulmonary veins); and (c) a basilar zone, extending from the inferior pulmonary veins to the base of the lungs. This method was initially proposed as an approach for evaluating patients presenting with hemoptysis using sequential axial images (29) and is easily adapted to helical scanning. Emphasizing adaptability, individual axial or helical scans, or variable combinations of both, can be obtained through these zones, allowing optimization of data acquisition. In those cases for which intravenous contrast is indicated, administration may be optimized by timing the bolus to coincide with scans from a particular zone, such as through the hilum in patients presenting with lobar and/ or segmental atelectasis (30).

It is axiomatic that optimal technique requires scan collimation that corresponds to the size of the airways to be evaluated. For the central airways this means that, at a minimum, 5-mm-thick sections must be obtained, with 3-mm collimation reserved for patients with possible occult neoplasm (1,31). Relatively thin, 5-mm scans are also valuable for assessing hilar pathology. Although optimal evaluation of the peripheral airways traditionally has required the use of 1-mm high-resolution computed tomography (HRCT) technique, in select cases helically acquired 3-mm sections may offer advantages, particularly for detecting subtle lack of bronchial tapering (32). Scans obtained in both deep inspiration and expiration also can be obtained either at a single level or through preselected regions, allowing physiologic evaluation of the tracheobronchial tree as well as the identification of areas of focal or diffuse air-trapping (33).

Retrospective Reconstruction Techniques

Although routine axial images remain the standard for identifying airways disease, these suffer important limitations, including (a) inability to identify mucosal disease; (b) limited accuracy in identifying submucosal disease, especially central extension of neoplasm; (c) limited accuracy in the estimation of length of tracheal and bronchial stenoses, and (d) limited assessment of obliquely coursing airways (6).

With the introduction of helical CT a variety of high-quality reconstruction techniques are now routinely available, including (a) multiplanar reconstructions (MPRs), including the use of curved multiplanar reformations; (b) multiplanar volume reconstructions (MPVRs), which involve the use of average-, maximum-, or minimum-intensity projection imaging; (c) external rendering with three-dimensional shaded surface displays; and (d) internal rendering, using either internal three-dimensional shaded surface reconstructions or volumetric rendering techniques to simulate the endoluminal appearance of airways—so-called virtual bronchoscopy (34–36).

Multiplanar Reconstructions

The most helpful of the potential reconstruction techniques currently available, MPRs should be obtained in any case for which the extent of airway pathology is not clearly determined on axial images (34). To date, external rendering and MPVRs have proved cumbersome and offer little additional value over MPRs (35). Multiplanar reconstructions are typically one-voxel-thick two-dimensional "tomographic" sections interpolated along an arbitrary plane or curved surface. Thicker sections using more than one pixel may also be obtained and often have the advantage of a smoother appearance. With conventional CT, MPRs were of limited value because of the prolonged imaging times needed to acquire a sufficient number of sections to generate quality reconstructions. These difficulties have been largely overcome with helical CT. MPRs also have the considerable advantage of computational efficiency, requiring only a few seconds to reconstruct with instantaneous window width and level manipulation. It is now possible to interactively obtain a series of single oblique reconstructions derived from corresponding axial sections, allowing individual airways to be displayed to best advantage along their nearest long axes.

Clinically, MPRs have proved of greatest value for evaluating focal airway stenoses, especially in patients following lung transplantation, or prolonged intubation (34). MPRs have also been shown to be of value in select patients with central lung cancer (36). In this setting, MPRs may allow more precise visualization of airway involvement as well as more accurate assessment of the peribronchial and/or mediastinal extent of disease.

Internal Rendering

Popularly referred to as virtual bronchoscopy, internal rendering can be performed using either volumetric or three-dimensional surface shaded reconstructions (35). Internal rendering allows visualization of the airways internally from a point source at a finite distance, simulating human perspective as seen through a bronchoscope. Images are then viewed through the tip of a cone with either a narrow (15-degree) or wide (60-degree) field of view. A flight path of sequential images can also be constructed and navigated either sequentially or in a cine loop, further simulating endoscopy.

Despite initial enthusiasm, a number of important limitations currently limit practical application. Endoluminal imaging, regardless of technique, is extremely time-consuming and currently requires specialized computers. More important, insufficient clinical data are available to judge the efficacy of endoluminal imaging. Speculation on possible clinical applications of "virtual bronchoscopy" has focused primarily on a potential role in the screening of patients with occult malignancy or as a guide bronchoscopy (38). However, the time necessary to generate or navigate these images currently precludes use as a screening test; in addition, the sensitivity of this technique has not been established and may be insufficient to ever obviate fiberoptic bronchoscopy.

CLINICAL APPLICATIONS

Bronchiectasis

Although routine HRCT remains most accurate for assessing peripheral airway disease, several recent reports do confirm a role for volumetric data acquisition, volumetric CT (VCT)

(32,39,40). In the most definitive study performed to date, Lucidarme and colleagues showed that use of 3-mm scans reconstructed every 2 mm (pitch = 1.6) was more accurate than routine HRCT in the identification of bronchiectasis despite the use of thicker sections (32). Surprisingly, although no patient had a diagnosis established solely by HRCT, in several cases, especially those with middle lobe disease, bronchiectasis was established solely by VCT. These data suggest that VCT is of value in patients in whom there is a high degree of clinical suspicion of bronchiectasis (i.e., patients with chronic productive cough or hemoptysis) if the initial HRCT examination is negative. This technique is of particular value for identifying subtle lack of peripheral tapering.

Occult Disease/Hemoptysis

Surprisingly, despite significant recent improvements in both endoscopic and CT technology, the etiology of hemoptysis often still proves elusive, with nearly 50% of cases remaining undiagnosed despite radiographic and bronchoscopic evaluation. As a result, there is little consensus concerning optimal diagnostic assessment (41). Current evidence suggests that CT plays an important role in evaluating these patients, especially those with nonlocalizing chest radiographs, provided care is taken to optimize scan technique (42). Our current protocol is based on the assumption that in most cases, clinically significant hemoptysis results either from a central endobronchial lesion or from peripheral bronchiectasis (41,42).

Even prior to the introduction of helical CT, a number of studies have validated a role for CT in assessing patients with hemoptysis. Millar and colleagues found that CT prospectively disclosed abnormalities in 50% of patients in whom chest radiographs and fiber optic bronchoscopy (FOB) proved nondiagnostic (43). Set and colleagues prospectively studied 91 patients with both CT and bronchoscopy and found that CT demonstrated all tumors seen by FOB as well as seven additional lesions, five of which were beyond the range of bronchoscopy (44). Most recently, McGuinness and colleagues prospectively studied 57 consecutive patients presenting with hemoptysis evaluated with both CT and FOB; they found that CT identified all cancers. Furthermore, the overall diagnostic yield of bronchoscopy was documented to be less than that with CT (47% compared with 61%) (41). It may be anticipated that with the introduction of newer helical CT techniques the reliability of CT to prospectively assess patients presenting with hemoptysis will substantially improve, rendering CT an important screening modality in these cases.

PARENCHYMAL DISEASE

Focal Lung Disease

Nodule Detection

From the time of its introduction it has been appreciated that helical scanning enhances the detection of pulmonary nodules, provided (as established by Kalender and colleagues in a study of phantom spheres of arbitrary diameter and contrast) overlapping sections are obtained (45). This is because optimal contrast and spatial resolution in conventional CT studies require that nodules be precisely centered in the plane of the section, whereas the contrast and spatial resolution of overlapping helical images may improve small lesion contrast by as much as a factor of 1.8. For those cases in which the main focus is nodule detection (e.g., patients with suspected pulmonary metastases), optimal results require that no more than 20% to 30% overlap be acquired (5).

Nodule Characterization

Compared with conventional thin-section HRCT, helical scanning ensures that contiguous scans will be obtained through the centers of individual nodules, of particular value in less than cooperative patients with small nodules. In this setting, a single acquisition suffices to ensure that images are obtained through the center of lesions. This is especially important when attempting to identify the presence of fat, as even minor degrees of partial volume averaging may result in an erroneous diagnosis (46). As important, helical acquisition allows for more precise evaluation of contrast enhancement within nodules. As recently documented by Swenson and colleagues, patterns of contrast enhancement within nodules may be predictive of benign versus malignant disease (47). Following a bolus of 100 mL of intravenous contrast media injected at a constant rate of 2 mL/sec, with images obtained 1, 2, 3, and 4 min, nonmalignant nodules almost always fail to enhance more than 20 HU. In distinction, almost all malignant nodules (as well as a substantial number of benign lesions) enhance more than 20 HU contrast enhancement (47). The potential advantages of helical scanning in this setting include (a) assurance that scans are obtained through nodules that otherwise may have been missed due to variations in respiration; (b) confidence that sections are obtained through the center of the nodule; and (c) optimization of comparison between scans taken at different times by allowing more precise identification of sections obtained at precisely the same level. In addition, and perhaps most important, helical acquisition allows more exact evaluation of the quality of the contrast bolus, an important consideration when attempting to measure contrast enhancement. It should be apparent that poor bolus administration may lead to the erroneous conclusion of an absence of nodule enhancement.

Diffuse Lung Disease

Technique

Diffuse infiltrative lung disease (DILD) is best evaluated with high-resolution CT technique (48). Because this requires thin (1–2-mm-thick) sections, helical scanning has to date played a small role in the evaluation of these cases (49,50). Although there is still no generally agreed-upon standard HRCT technique, most investigators agree that by definition HRCT requires (1) the use of thin collimation and (2) image reconstruction with a high spatial frequency (sharp) algorithm. Although in most cases optimal images require increasing kilovolt peak (kVp) or mA, it has been documented that clinically useful images may be obtained with a low-dose technique with mA as low as 40. Recent studies assessing the lung-parenchyma-comparing routine with low-dose (20–80 mA) HRCT techniques have concluded that in most cases low-dose techniques prove roughly equivalent for assessing the lungs (51). In our judgment, low-dose scans are indicated for pediatric populations and for younger adults when repeated follow-up CT scanning can be predicted. In addition to these factors, it should be noted that for most HRCT protocols, scans are routinely obtained only with patients in the supine position at end-inspiratory lung volume. Prone images are reserved for only patients with suspected basilar lung disease, where supine images are nondiagnostic because of dependent lung density, a frequent normal variant.

Scan Protocols

Although there is general agreement on the parameters necessary for optimizing individual slices, there is little agreement about how many images should be obtained to qualify as a high-resolution CT study (48). Two fundamentally different approaches to HRCT have been used. The first is to obtain only few HRCT images through select regions of interest as part of a general survey examination of the chest. Although this approach is adequate when a general survey of the thorax is indicated, this does not qualify as a true HRCT study if the clinical indication for the study is DILD.

The second approach is to obtain HRCT images only, in lieu of performing a conventional CT examination. Our current practice is to obtain 1–1.5-mm sections every 1 cm from the lung apices to the diaphragms. This ensures adequate uniform sampling of all lung zones. In patients suspected of having airways or obstructive disease on the basis of clinical pulmonary function or of plain radiographic findings, or in those found to have so-called mosaic attenuation on initial HRCT images, it has been recommended that a few select additional images be obtained with end expiratory lung volume in order to detect focal areas of air-trapping (33). Expiratory scans at three selected levels (aortic arch, hila, lower lobes) are generally sufficient for showing significant air-trapping when present; alternatively, expiratory images may be obtained in select regions of interest predetermined from initial inspiratory HRCT images.

REFERENCES

1. Kalender WA, Seissler W, Klotz E, Vock P. Spiral volumetric CT with single-breath-hold technique, continuous transport, and continuous scanner rotation. *Radiology* 1990;176:181–183.
2. Costello P, Anderson W, Blume D. Pulmonary nodule: evaluation with spiral volumetric CT. *Radiology* 1991; 179:875–876.
3. Costello P, Ecker CP, Tello R, Hartnell GG. Assessment of the thoracic aorta by spiral CT. *AJR* 1992;158: 1127–1130.
4. Naidich DP. Helical computed tomography of the thorax. Clinical applications. *Radiol Clin North Am* 1994; 32:759–774.
5. Brink JA. Technical aspects of helical (spiral) CT. *Radiol Clin North Am* 1995;33:825.
6. Naidich DP, Gruden JF, McGuinness G, McCauley DI, Bhalla M. Volumetric (helical/spiral) CT (VCT) of the airways. *J Thorac Imag* 1997;12:11–28.
7. Costello P, Dupuy DE, Ecker CP, Tello R. Spiral CT of the thorax with reduced volume of contrast material: a comparative study. *Radiology* 1992;183:663–666.
8. Rubin GD, Lane MJ, Bloch DA, Leung AN, Stark P. Optimization of thoracic spiral CT: effects of iodinated contrast medium concentration. *Radiology* 1996;201:785–791.
9. Schnyder P, Meuli R, Wicky S. Injection techniques. In: M Rémy-Jardin and J Rémy, eds. *Spiral CT of the chest.* Berlin: Springer-Verlag, 1996;Chapter 4.
10. Silverman P, Roberts S, Tiffl MC, Brown B, Fox SH. Helical CT of the liver: clinical application of a computer automated scanning technique—Smartprep—for obtaining images with optimal contrast enhancement. *AJR* 1995;165:73–78.
11. Rémy-Jardin M, Rémy J, Wattinne L, Giraud F. Central pulmonary thromboembolism: diagnosis with spiral volumetric CT with the single-breath-hold technique. Comparison with pulmonary angiography. *Radiology* 1992;185:381–387.
12. Rémy-Jardin M, Rémy J, Deschildre F, et al. Diagnosis of pulmonary embolism with spiral CT: comparison with pulmonary angiography and scintigraphy. *Radiology* 1996;200:699–706.
13. Sinner WN. Computed tomography of pulmonary thromboembolism. *Eur J Radiol* 1982;2:8–13.
14. Rémy-Jardin M, Duyck P, Rémy J, et al. Hilar lymph nodes: identification with spiral CT and histologic correlation. *Radiology* 1995;196:387–394.
15. Rémy-Jardin M, Rémy J, Cauvain O, Petyt L, Wannebroucq J, Beregi J-P. Diagnosis of central pulmonary embolism with helical CT: role of two-dimensional multiplanar reformations. *AJR* 1995;165:1131–1138.
16. Hull RE, Hirsch J, Carter CJ, et al. Pulmonary angiography, ventilation lung scanning, and venography for clinically suspected pulmonary embolism with abnormal perfusion lung scan. *Ann Intern Med* 1983;98:891–899.
17. Teigen CL, Maus TP, Sheedy PF, et al. Pulmonary embolism: diagnosis with contrast-enhanced electron-beam CT and comparison with pulmonary angiography. *Radiology* 1995;194:313–319.
18. Schwickert HC, Kauczor HE, Schweden FJ, Thelen M. Mosaic oligemia in CT of patients with chronic pulmonary embolism: correlation with the diameter of the feeding pulmonary artery. *Radiology* 1995;197(P):303.
19. Schmidt HC, Kauczor HU, Schild HH, et al. Pulmonary hypertension in patients with chronic pulmonary thromboembolism: chest radiograph and CT evaluation before and after surgery. *European Radiol* 1996;6: 817–825.
20. Zeman RK, Berman PM, Silverman PM, et al. Diagnosis of aortic dissection: value of helical CT with multiplanar reformation and three-dimensional rendering. *AJR* 1995;164:1375–1380.

21. Williams DM, Joshi A, Dake MD, Deeb CM, Miller DC, Abrams GD. Aortic cobwebs: an anatomic marker identifying the false lumen in aortic dissection—imaging and pathologic correlation. *Radiology* 1994;190: 167–174.
22. Quint LE, Francis IR, Williams DM, et al. Evaluation of thoracic aortic disease with the use of helical CT and multiplanar reconstructions: comparison with surgical findings. *Radiology* 1996;201:37–41.
23. Burns MA, Molina PL, Gutierrez ER, et al. Motion artifact simulating aortic dissection on CT. *AJR* 1991;157: 465–467.
24. Chung JW, Park JH, Im J-G, Chung MJ, Han MC, Ahn H. Spiral CT angiography of the thoracic aorta. *Radiographics* 1996;1996:811–824.
25. Kopecky KK, Gokhale HS, Hawes DR. Spiral CT angiography of the aorta. *Semin Ultrasound CT MR* 1996; 17:304–315.
26. Sommer T, Fehske W, Holzknecht N, et al. Aortic dissection: a comparative study of diagnosis with spiral CT, multiplanar transesophageal echocardiography, and MR imaging. *Radiology* 1996;199:347–352.
27. Rubin GD, Dake MD, Semba CP. Current status of three-dimensional spiral CT scanning for imaging the vasculature. *Radiol Clin North Am* 1995;33:51–70.
28. Sartorettischefer S, Sartoretti C, Kotulek T, Vollrath T. Atherosclerotic penetrating ulcer of the aorta: typical morphology on CT. A review of five cases. *Eur Radiol* 1995;5:657–662.
29. Naidich DP, Harkin TJ. Airways and lung: correlation of CT with fiberoptic bronchoscopy. *Radiology* 1995; 197:1–12.
30. Glazer HS, Anderson DJ, Sagel SS. Bronchial impaction in lobar collapse: CT demonstration and pathologic correlation. *AJR* 1989;153:485–488.
31. Heiken JP, Brink JA, Vannier MW. Spiral (helical) CT. *Radiology* 1993;189:647–656.
32. Lucidarme O, Grenier P, Coche E, Lenoir S, Aubert B, Beigelman C. Bronchiectasis: comparative assessment with thin-section CT and helical CT. *Radiology* 1996;200:673–679.
33. Webb WR, Stern EJ, Kanth N, Gamsu G. Dynamic pulmonary CT: findings in normal adult men. *Radiology* 1993;186:117–124.
34. Quint LE, Whyte RI, Kazerooni EA, et al. Stenosis of the central airways: evaluation by using helical CT with multiplanar reconstructions. *Radiology* 1995;194:871–877.
35. Rubin GD, Napel S, Leung AN. Editorial. Volumetric analysis of volumetric data: achieving a paradigm shift. *Radiology* 1996;200:312–317.
36. Vining DJ, Liu K, Choplin RH, Haponik EF. Virtual bronchoscopy: relationships of virtual reality endobronchial simulations to actual bronchoscopic findings. *Chest* 1996;109:549–553.
37. Kauczor H-U, Wolcke B, Fischer B, Mildenberger P, Lorenz J, Thelen M. Three-dimensional helical CT of the tracheobronchial tree: evaluation of imaging protocols and assessment of suspected stenoses with bronchoscopic correlation. *AJR* 1996;167:419–424.
38. Quint LE, McShan DL, Glazer GM, Orringer MB, Francis IR, Gross BH. Three-dimensional CT of central lung tumors. *Clin Imaging* 1990;14:323–329.
39. Van der Bruggen-Bogaartw BAHA, van der Bruggen HMJG, van Waes PFGM, Lammers J-WJ. Assessment of bronchiectasis: comparison of HRCT and spiral volumetric CT. *JCAT* 1996;20:15–19.
40. Engeler CE, Tashjian JH, Engeler CM, Geise RA, Holm JC, Ritenour ER. Volumetric high-resolution CT in the diagnosis of interstitial lung disease and bronchiectasis: diagnostic accuracy and radiation dose. *AJR* 1993; 163:31–35.
41. McGuinness G, Beacher JR, Harkin TJ, Garay SM, Rom WN, Naidich DP. Hemoptysis: prospective high-resolution CT/bronchoscopic correlation. *Chest* 1994;105(4):1155–1162.
42. Marshall TJ, Flower CDR, Jackson JE. The role of radiology in the investigation and management of patients with haemoptysis. *Clin Radiol* 1996;51:391–400.
43. Millar A, Boothroyd A, Edwards D, Hetzel M. The role of computed tomography (CT) in the investigation of unexplained hemoptysis. *Resp Med* 1992;86:39–44.
44. Set PAK, Flower CDR, Smith IE, Cahn AP, Twentyman OP, Shneerson JM. Hemoptysis: comparative study of the role of CT and fiberoptic bronchoscopy. *Radiology* 1993;189:677–680.
45. Kalender WA, Polacin A, Suss C. A comparison of conventional and spiral CT: an experimental study on the detection of spherical lesions. *J Comput Assist Tomogr* 1994;18:167–176.
46. Siegelman SS, Khouri NF, Scott WW, et al. Pulmonary hamartoma: CT findings. *Radiology* 1986;160:313–317.
47. Swenson SJ, Brown LR, Colby TV, Weaver AL. Pulmonary nodules: CT evaluation of enhancement with iodinated contrast material. *Radiology* 1995;194:393–398.
48. Webb WR, Müller NL, Naidich DP. *High resolution CT of the lung.* Philadelphia: Lippincott-Raven, 1996.
49. Bhalla M, Naidich DP, McGuinness G, Gruden JF, Leitman BS, McCauley DI. Diffuse lung disease: assessment with helical CT-preliminary observations of the role of maximum and minimum projection images. *Radiology* 1996;200:341–347.
50. Rémy-Jardin M, Rémy J, Artaud D, Deschildre F, Duhamel A. Diffuse infiltrative lung disease: clinical value of sliding-thin-slab maximum intensity projection CT scans in the detection of mild micronodular patterns. *Radiology* 1996;200:333–339.
51. Zwirewich CV, Mayo JR, Müller NL. Low-dose high-resolution CT of lung parenchyma. *Radiology* 1991;180: 413–417.

Protocol 1:
THORACIC SURVEY (Fig. 1)

INDICATION:	*Detection/Staging thoracic neoplasia/ complex pulmonary-pleural disease*
SCANNER SETTINGS:	kVp: 120 mAs: 250
PHASE OF RESPIRATION:	Suspended inspiration ($\pm$) hyperventilation
SLICE THICKNESS:	5–10 mm
PITCH:	1.0–2.0 (Variable pitch $>$ 1 recommended in larger patients to cover the adrenals if images acquired only in a single breath-hold. *Important:* If a pitch of more than 1 is used, then collimation should be reduced so that effective slice thickness is 7–8 mm maximally.)
HELICAL EXPOSURE TIME:	Single and/or multiple sequential acquisitions with variable breath-hold periods
RECONSTRUCTION INTERVAL:	5–10 mm
SUPERIOR EXTENT:	Superior margin of clavicles (above lung apices)
INFERIOR EXTENT:	Posterior costophrenic sulci (caudal lung bases)

IV CONTRAST:	Concentration:	LOCM 300–320 mg I/mL or HOCM 282 mg I/mL (60% solution)
Low-Volume Technique:	Rate:	2 mL/sec for 20 sec (40 mL) followed by 1 mL/sec for 20 sec (20 mL)
	Scan Delay:	20 sec
	Total Volume:	60 mL
Standard-Volume Technique:	Rate:	3 mL/sec
	Scan Delay:	15–20 sec or computer automated scanning technology (CAST)/ bolus care
	Total Volume:	100–125 mL

COMMENTS

1. The low-volume technique should be used when there is concern regarding the patient's total dose of IV contrast media (e.g., renal function, potential arteriography).
2. Most centers examine the upper abdomen after the chest during the portal venous phase. A 15-sec interval may be set between the two acquisitions, allowing the patient to breathe.
3. Abdominal parameters are 8-mm collimation, pitch 1, 120 kV, 280–320 mA. Reconstructed at 8-mm intervals with standard algorithm. See Chapter 3 for full protocol.
4. In those cases in which radiation exposure is a concern, (especially younger patients), survey images of the lungs and airways, in particular, may be obtained with a low-dose technique using 40–80 mA for the lung parenchyma.

FIG. 1. (**A**) Transverse scan through the carina confirms the presence of an inhomogeneous right-upper-lobe mass consistent with bronchogenic carcinoma (T) with a large precarinal lymph node (*arrow*) (8-mm collimation, pitch 1.2). (**B**) Abdominal examination using the same-contrast bolus after a 15-sec interscan delay between thorax and abdomen. Two 1-cm low-attenuation areas are seen in the liver (*arrows*) consistent with metastases.

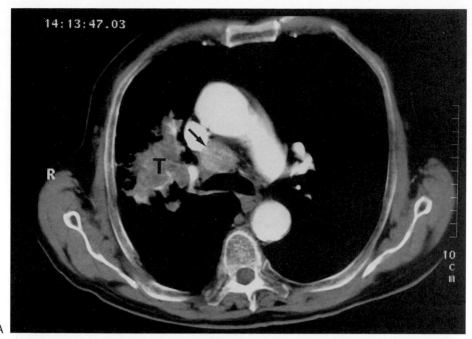

A

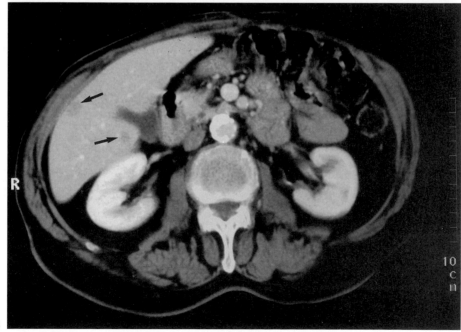

B

Protocol 2:
NECK/THORACIC INLET (Fig. 2)

INDICATION: *Combined study; head/neck tumors; suspected superior vena cava syndrome, vocal cord paralysis, brachial plexus*

SCANNER SETTINGS:

	Neck	Chest
kVp:	140	120
mAs:	250	250

PHASE OF RESPIRATION:

Neck imaging:	Quiet breathing or suspended inspiration
Chest imaging:	Suspended inspiration

SLICE THICKNESS:

Neck:	3–5 mm parallel to the cords, neck positioning
Chest:	7–8 mm

PITCH: 1.0–2.0, effective slice thickness as with all thorax cases should be 7–8 mm maximally and 3–5 mm for the neck unless large masses.

HELICAL EXPOSURE TIME: Consecutive breath-hold acquisitions with interscan delay of 12–15 sec (neck to chest) allowing for breathing.

RECONSTRUCT INTERVAL: 2–4 mm for the neck; 6–7 mm for the thoracic inlet

SUPERIOR EXTENT: Base of the tongue

INFERIOR EXTENT: Carina

IV CONTRAST:

Concentration:	LOCM 300–320 mg I/mL or HOCM 282 mg I/mL (60% solution)
Scan Delay:	15 sec
Rate:	2 mL/sec
Total Volume:	120–150 mL

COMMENTS:
1. Study may be extended to include the entire thorax to the diaphragms as clinically indicated.
2. In cases for which multiplanar or three-dimensional reconstructions or internal rendering is planned it is necessary to maintain identical collimation, field of view and scan coordinates for each acquisition.

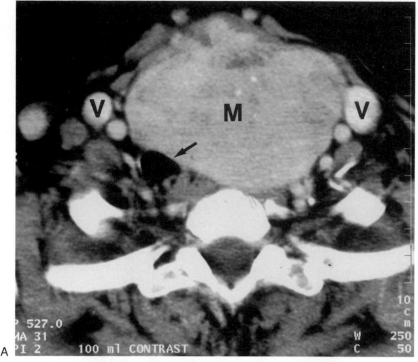

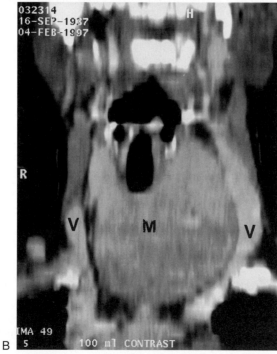

FIG. 2. (**A**) Markedly enhancing mass (M) arising from the thyroid displacing the trachea to the right (*arrow*) (A) jugular veins (V). (**B**) Coronal multiplanar reconstruction (MPR) through the mass shows lateral displacement of the jugular veins (V) by a multinodular goiter (M).

Protocol 3:
PULMONARY EMBOLI (Fig. 3)

INDICATION:	*Acute or chronic*
SCANNER SETTINGS:	kVp: 140 mAs: 210
PHASE OF RESPIRATION:	Suspended expiration
SLICE THICKNESS:	3 mm
PITCH:	1.6–2.0
HELICAL EXPOSURE TIME:	Single breath-hold period
RECONSTRUCTION INTERVAL:	2 mm
SUPERIOR EXTENT:	Top of aortic arch
INFERIOR EXTENT:	Interior pulmonary veins as a minimum

IV CONTRAST:

Concentration:	**A.** LOCM 300–320 mg I/mL at 3 mL/sec **B.** LOCM 150 mg I/mL (30% solution) at 4 mL/sec
Scan Delay:	Timed bolus following initial test injection of 20 mL of contrast followed by images every 10 sec strongly recommended to optimize visualization of the pulmonary arteries; or 15–20-sec delay
Total Volume:	150 mL (to include initial 20 mL test dose)

COMMENTS:

1. Patients need to breath-hold without a Valsalva maneuver.
2. Protocol B uses more dilute contrast at a higher flow rate to prevent streak artifacts from contrast in the superior vena cava.
3. Images should be displayed on narrow and wide window settings to distinguish arteries from veins.
4. MPRs of vessels obliquely oriented can be imaged along their longitudinal axis assisting differentiation between intraluminal clot and extrinsic hilar compression.

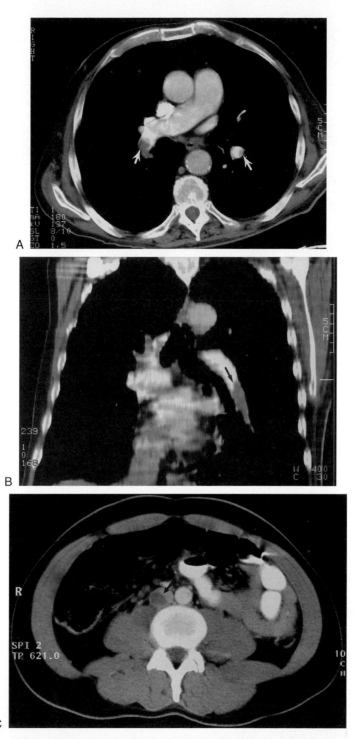

FIG. 3. (**A**) Note bilateral lower lobar emboli (*arrows*). (**B**) Oblique multiplanar reconstruction through the left lower lobe pulmonary artery confirms the presence of clot in the left lower lobe pulmonary artery (*arrow*). (**C**) Note large thrombus also seen in the interior vena cava (*arrow*).

Protocol 4:
THORACIC AORTA (Fig. 4)

INDICATION: *Aortic dissection, aneurysm assessment,
penetrating aortic ulcer*

SCANNER SETTINGS: kVp: 120
mAs: 250

PHASE OF RESPIRATION: Suspended inspiration

SLICE THICKNESS: 5–8 mm

PITCH: 1.6–2.0

HELICAL EXPOSURE TIME: Single and/or multiple breath-holds, 10–15 sec
interscan delay as clinically indicated

**RECONSTRUCTION
  INTERVAL:**   4–6 mm

SUPERIOR EXTENT: 3 cm above aortic arch

INFERIOR EXTENT: To the diaphragm: continue caudally if dissection
extends into abdominal aorta.

IV CONTRAST:

Concentration:	LOCM 300–320 mg I/mL or HOCM 282 mg I/mL (60% solution)
Rate:	3–4 mL/sec (use computer automated scanning technology [CAST] or a test injection)
Scan Delay:	See suggestions for pulmonary emboli in Protocol 3.
Volume:	120–150 mL

COMMENTS:

1. Initial noncontrast scans at the level of the arch and mid-ascending aorta as a minimum should be obtained in all cases to identify patients with acute intramural hematomas and/or displaced intimal calcifications
2. Retrospective or prospective segmentation may be useful to avoid pitfall of motion at the aortic root. This pulsatile artifact has been reported when scans are performed in less than 1.5 sec. Alternatively, axial clusters can be performed with a 2-sec scan time to avoid this pitfall immediately following helical scans.

3. With abdominal extension of dissections or aneurysms, collimation can be increased to 5–8 mm with a pitch of 2 providing coverage to the aortic bifurcation.
4. Multiplanar two-dimensional reconstructions assist display of the dissecting membrane and the true and false lumina.

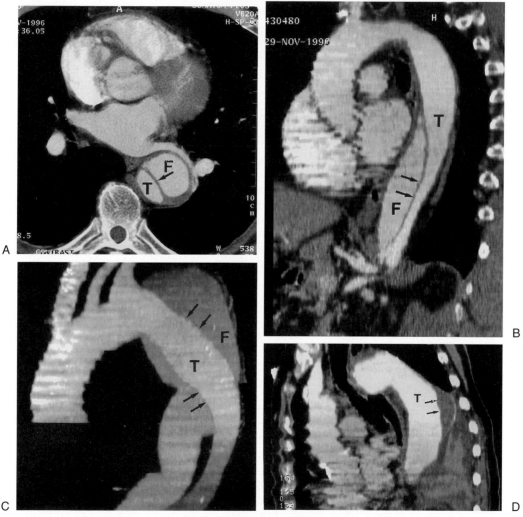

FIG. 4. (**A**) Axial scan shows clear delineation of the intimal flap, type B dissection (*arrow*), and true (T) and false (F) lumens. (**B**) Curved planar reconstruction through the aorta shows the clear delineation of the compressed true lumen (T), intimal flap (*arrows*) and false lumen (F). (**C**) Maximum-intensity projection image of a different patient with a type B aortic dissection shows the denser true (T) lumen (*arrows*) and the less dense false (F) lumen extending up to the origin of the left subclavian artery. (**D**) Sagittal reconstruction through the descending thoracic aorta (of a different patient with an atherosclerotic aortic aneurysm) shows calcification in the aortic wall, mural thrombus (*arrows*), and contrast-filled true (T) lumen.

Protocol 5:
AIRWAY DISEASE (Fig. 5)

INDICATION: *Bronchiectasis, inflammatory disease, endobronchial lesions*

SCANNER SETTINGS: kVp: 120
mAs: 250

PHASE OF RESPIRATION: Suspended inspiration ($\pm$) hyperventilation

SLICE THICKNESS: 1–3 mm

PITCH: 1.0–2.0

HELICAL EXPOSURE TIME: Multiple sequential acquisitions

RECONSTRUCTION INTERVAL: Every 2–3 mm

SUPERIOR EXTENT: Thoracic inlet

INFERIOR EXTENT: Lung bases

PHASE ACQUISITION:
1. Initial 1-mm routine axial HRCT images reconstructed every 10 mm from the thoracic inlet to 2 cm above the carina, followed by:
2. 3-mm sections through the inferior pulmonary veins; and then:
3. 1 mm routine axial high-resolution (HRCT) images reconstructed every 10 mm to the lung bases

IV CONTRAST: None

COMMENTS:
1. This protocol represents a modification of a standard high-resolution CT protocol for evaluating bronchiectasis, adapted for helical scan acquisition.
2. Three-mm collimation (pitch = 2.0; reconstruction interval = 2 mm) preferred for detecting subtle central endobronchial pathology.
3. Although 1-mm sections through the lung bases remains the standard for detecting basilar bronchiectasis, these may be substituted by 3-mm sections.
4. Use high spatial resolution reconstruction (bone) algorithm.
5. Additional images also may be obtained in deep expiration to differentiate between focal areas of groundglass attenuation due to focal air-trapping from mosaic perfusion.
6. Gantry angulation should be considered in select cases, especially those involving the middle lobe or lingula airways to decrease volume-averaging artifacts.

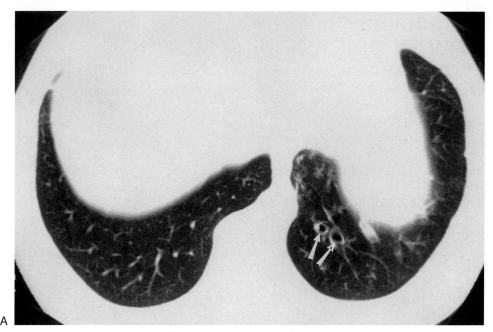

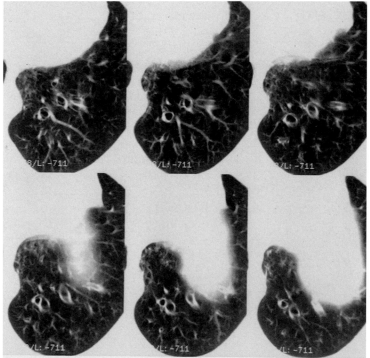

FIG. 5. Bronchiectasis: evaluation with helical CT. (**A**) One-mm routine axial CT section through the lung bases demonstrates dilated peripheral bronchi (*arrows*) in the posterobasilar segment of the left lower lobe. (**B**). Enlargements of sequential 3-mm helical sections reconstructed every 2 mm obtained through the same anatomic region of the left lower lobe as shown in **A**, using a pitch of 2. In comparison to routine axial images, volumetric acquisition allows each individual airway to be evaluated sequentially as it extends toward the periphery. This is especially important in cases where the primary abnormality is a lack of tapering.

Protocol 6:
AIRWAY DISEASE (Fig. 6)

INDICATION:	*Occult airway disease (hemoptysis)*
SCANNER SETTINGS:	kVp: 120
	mAs: 250
PHASE OF RESPIRATION:	Suspended inspiration ($\pm$) hyperventilation
SLICE THICKNESS:	3–5 mm
PITCH:	1.0–2.0
HELICAL EXPOSURE TIME:	Multiple sequential acquisitions
RECONSTRUCTion INTERVAL:	Every 2–3 mm
SUPERIOR EXTENT:	True vocal cords
INFERIOR EXTENT:	Lung bases
PHASE ACQUISTION:	1. Initial 3–5-mm sections from the level of the true cords (C5) to 2 cm above the carina, followed by:
	2. Three-mm sections at a minimum through the inferior pulmonary veins; and then:
	3. One-mm routine axial HRCT images every 10 mm to the lung bases.

IV CONTRAST:

OPTIONAL	
Concentration:	LOCM 300–320 mg I/mL or HOCM 282 mg I/mL (60% solution) at 3 mL/sec or 150 mg I/mL (30% solution) at 4 mL/sec
Scan Delay:	15–20 sec
Total Volume:	100–125 mL

COMMENTS:

1. This protocol represents a modification of a standard high-resolution CT protocol for evaluating patients with hemoptysis designed to optimize identification of both endobronchial lesions and bronchiectasis.
2. Three-mm collimation (pitch = 2.0; reconstruction interval = 2 mm) preferred for detecting subtle central endobronchial pathology.
3. Although 1-mm sections through the lung bases remain the standard for detecting basilar bronchiectasis, these may be substituted by 3-mm sections
4. In cases for which multiplanar, three-dimensional or virtual endoscopic imaging is planned, it is necessary that each scan acquisition use the same field of view (FOV), collimation, and scan coordinates.
5. IV contrast may be administered either at the outset of the examination or selectively during any of the three phases, depending on the likely point of bronchial obstruction (see Protocol 6).
6. Use high spatial resolution reconstruction (bone) algorithm.
7. Gantry angulation should be considered in select cases, especially those involving the middle lobe or lingula airways to decrease volume-averaging artifacts.

FIG. 6. Endobronchial tumor—advantage of multiplanar reconstructions. (**A,B**) Identical 3-mm sections acquired helically through the mid-trachea imaged with lung (**A**) and mediastinal (**B**) windows, respectively, following the administration of a 100-mL bolus of IV contrast shows a well-defined intraluminal tumor mass (*arrow*) causing near complete obliteration of the tracheal lumen. Note that there is clear extension of the tumor mass into the adjacent mediastinal soft tissues without obvious invasion of adjacent vessels. (**C**) Coronal multiplanar reconstruction imaged with lung windows shows to advantage both the superior and inferior extent of tumor (*arrow*). (**D**) Oblique multiplanar reconstruction images with mediastinal windows shows the relationship between the tumor (t) and adjacent mediastinal soft tissues (*arrows*). In this case, despite mediastinal invasion, the aorta and left subclavian arteries are clearly uninvolved. Determination of the true endo- and extraluminal extent of tumor is critical for accurate presurgical assessment. In this case an adenoid cystic carcinoma was successfully resected.

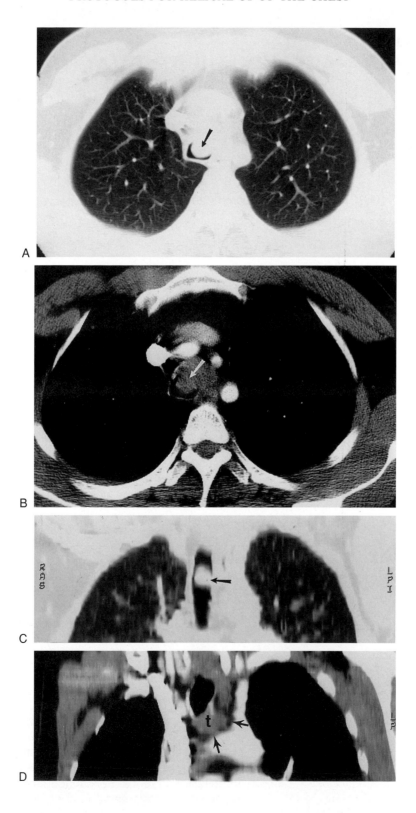

Protocol 7:
AIRWAY PATENCY, HILAR EVALUATION
(Figs. 7, 8)

INDICATION: *Atelectasis, stenoses, dehiscence, hilar masses*

SCANNER SETTINGS: kVp: 120
                                 mAs: 250

PHASE OF RESPIRATION: Suspended inspiration ($+$/-) hyperventilation

SLICE THICKNESS: 3–5 mm

PITCH: 1.0–2.0

HELICAL EXPOSURE TIME: Single and/or multiple sequential acquisitions as
                                 needed

**RECONSTRUCTION
 INTERVAL:**   Every 2–4 mm with 1–2 mm reconstruction
                                 interval optional through select regions of
                                 interest

SUPERIOR EXTENT: **SINGLE PHASE ACQUISITION:**
  thoracic inlet   5 mm sections (pitch = 2; reconstruction interval
                                   = 4 mm) from the thoracic inlet to the
                                   hemidiaphragms, or:

INFERIOR EXTENT: **3 PHASE ACQUISITION:**
  lung bases   1. Initial 5 mm sections from the apices to 2 cm
                                    above the carina, followed by:
                                 2. 3–5 mm sections through the inferior
                                    pulmonary veins, and then:
                                 3. 5 mm sections to the level of the diaphragms

IV CONTRAST:

OPTIONAL	
Concentration:	LOCM 300–320 mg I/mL or HOCM 282 mg I/mL (60%solution) at 3 mL/sec or 150 mg I/mL (30% solution) at 4 mL/sec
Scan Delay:	15–20 sec
Total Volume:	100–125 mL

COMMENTS: 1. 3-mm collimation (pitch = 2.0; reconstruction
                                    interval = 2 mm) preferred in those cases for
                                    which precise location of lesion/obstruction is
                                    known.
                                 2. If multiple sequential helical acquisitions are
                                    obtained, maintain same field of view (FOV)

and scan coordinates and collimation if either multiplanar, three-dimensional, or virtual endoscopic reconstructions are planned.

3. IV contrast may be administered either at the outset of the examination or selectively during any of the three phases depending on the likely point of bronchial obstruction.

4. Use high spatial resolution reconstruction (bone) algorithm.

5. Gantry angulation should be considered in select cases, especially those involving the middle lobe or lingula airways to decrease volume-averaging artifacts.

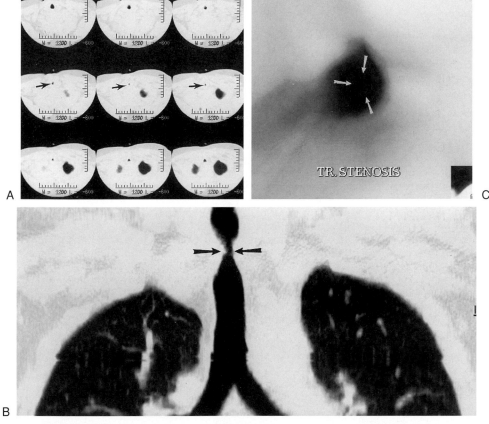

FIG. 7. Tracheal stenosis—evaluation with multiplanar reconstructions and internal rendering. (**A**) Sequential 3-mm sections acquired helically through the thoracic inlet show focal narrowing of the trachea (*arrows*). (**B**) Multiplanar reconstruction in the coronal plane shows to better advantage than corresponding axial reconstructions the true extent and severity of the stenosis (*arrows*). (**C**) Internal rendering of the stenosis (*arrows*) as seen from above—so-called virtual bronchoscopy--allows simulation of the endoscopic appearance of airway pathology.

FIG. 8. Hilar carcinoid—evaluation with sequential contrast-enhanced helical acquisitions. (**A**) Posteroanterior radiograph shows subtle density in the superior portion of the left hilum (*arrows*). (**B**) Enlargement of 3-mm section acquired helically through the left hilum shows left hilar mass (*arrows*), causing slight compression of the adjacent bronchus. This appearance could be confused with an enlarged hilar vessel. (**C**) Coronal multiplanar reconstruction shows to better advantage that this mass (*arrows*) is distinct from adjacent vessels. (**D–F**) Enlargements of 3-mm helical sections through the left hilum obtained 1, 2, and 4 min, respectively, following a bolus of 100 mL of 60% IV contrast medium. Note that the mean density within this lesion (shown at the bottom of each image) measures 186, 113, and 78 HU, respectively at 1, 2, and 4 min, indicative of considerable neovascularity, almost paralleling the adjacent pulmonary artery. This degree of enhancement within a central mass abutting a bronchus is characteristic of a carcinoid tumor, subsequently verified at surgery. The ability to acquire sequential helical data sets through the hilum allows optimization of contrast enhancement for assessing both hilar vessels as well as adjacent tumors.

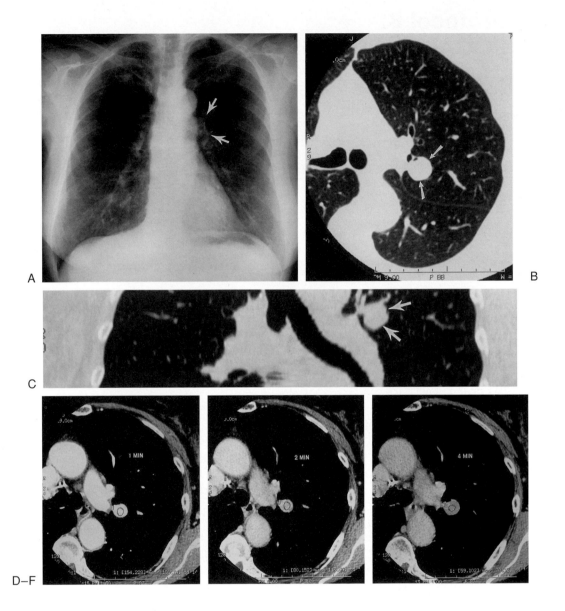

Protocol 8:
FOCAL LUNG DISEASE (Fig. 9)

INDICATION: *Solitary nodule/arteriovenous malformations*

SCANNER SETTINGS: kVp: 120
                            mAs: 250

PHASE OF RESPIRATION: Suspended inspiration

SLICE THICKNESS: 1–3 mm

PITCH: 1.0–2.0

HELICAL EXPOSURE TIME: Single breath-hold through region of interest
                            (ROI)

**RECONSTRUCTION
  INTERVAL:**   1–3 mm

SUPERIOR EXTENT: Above nodule

INFERIOR EXTENT: Below nodule

SECTION SEQUENCING: Following an initial thoracic survey, 1–3-mm
                            sections are obtained through a select ROI
                            (nodule) without contrast to assess for possible
                            calcification and/or fat. Sequence may be
                            repeated through more than one ROI, if
                            necessary.

IV CONTRAST: For cases in which nodule enhancement is to be
                            assessed, the following parameters are
                            recommended:

Concentration:	HOCM 282 mg I/mL (60% solution)
Rate:	2 mL/sec
Scan Acquisitions:	1, 2, 3, and 4 min
Total Volume:	100 mL
FOV:	19 cm centered on the nodule

COMMENTS:

1. Although of potential value in select cases, the use of a phantom for accurate CT densitometry is not requisite.
2. In those cases in which radiation exposure is a particular concern, initial survey images may be obtained with a low-dose technique using 40–80 mA.
3. A modification of this protocol also may be applied to patients with suspected arteriovenous malformations. In these cases a single acquisition 20 sec following a bolus of 125 mL of IV contrast using 3-mm collimation (pitch = 2.0; reconstruction interval = 2 mm) allows precise localization and morphologic characterization, including high-quality multiplanar and three-dimensional reconstructions. For smaller malformations and obliquely oriented vessels narrower collimation and intervals are needed to minimize partial volume effects.

---▶

FIG. 9. Solitary pulmonary nodules—helical CT evaluation. (**A**) One-mm noncontrast-enhanced CT section shows a well-defined solitary nodule (*arrow*) in the right lower lobe. The
mean density of this lesion measured within the range of fluid. (**B,C**) Enlargements of the same
3-mm section helically acquired 1 min following the bolus administration of 100 mL of 60%
iodinated contrast media, imaged with lung and mediastinal windows, respectively. These show
that a well-defined lesion abuts a branch of the superior segmental bronchus with a mean
density of only 12 HU. Similar density measurements were obtained at 2, 3, and 4 min, indicating
that this lesion is avascular (compare with Protocol 7, Fig. 8). These findings suggested the
possibility of an intraparenchymal cyst or abscess. (**D**) Section through this nodule obtained
at the time of transthoracic needle (*arrow*) aspiration (TTNA) shows accurate placement of the
tip of the needle. In our experience TTNA is much more easily performed with helical imaging
as images can be rapidly obtained through the tip of the needle in a single pass of the CT
scanner. Approximately 2 mL of clear sterile fluid were aspirated. At thoracotomy this lesion
proved to have cartilage in the wall, suggesting the diagnosis of an intrapulmonary bronchogenic cyst.

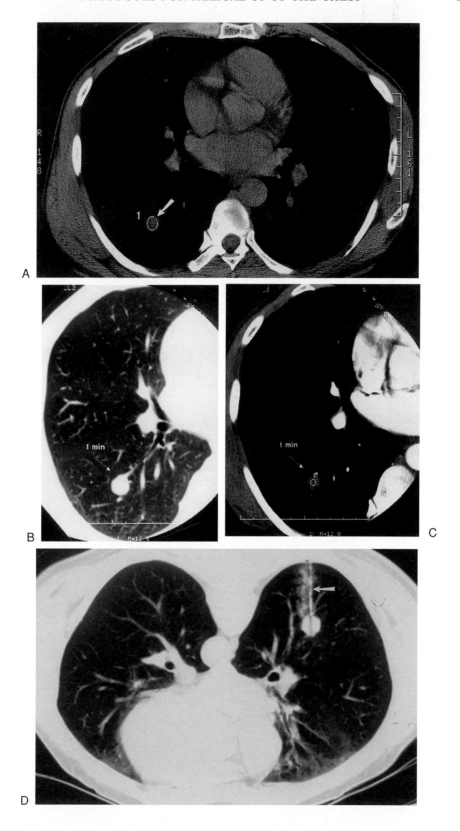

Protocol 9:
DIFFUSE INFILTRATIVE LUNG DISEASE: HIGH-RESOLUTION COMPUTED TOMOGRAPHY (HRCT) (Fig. 10)

INDICATION:	*Diffuse parenchymal lung disease characterization*
SCANNER SETTINGS:	kVp: 120–140 mAs: 200–250
PHASE OF RESPIRATION:	Suspended inspiration
SLICE THICKNESS:	1 mm (obtained every 1 cm)
PITCH:	1.0–2.0
EXPOSURE TIME:	Routine 1–2-sec scan time
SUPERIOR EXTENT:	Lung apices
INFERIOR EXTENT:	Lung bases
SECTION SEQUENCE:	Conventional 1-mm images from the lung apices to the diaphragms every 10 mm; ± 1-mm helical images through select ROI
IV CONTRAST:	None
COMMENTS:	1. A survey study of the entire thorax alternately can be performed with 1-mm sections obtained every 2–2.5 cm. 2. Additional images obtained prone may be of value in select cases with basilar parenchymal disease. 3. Additional images also may be obtained in deep expiration to differentiate between focal areas of groundglass attenuation due to focal air-trapping from mosaic perfusion.

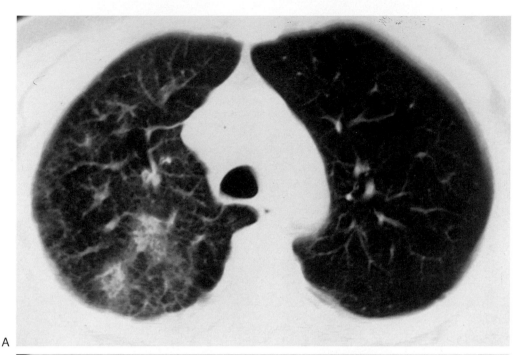

A

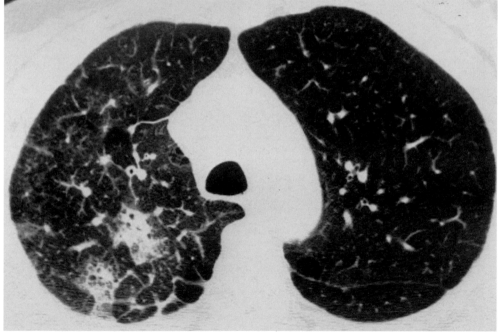

B

FIG. 10. Lymphangitic carcinomatosis: evaluation with standard- and high-resolution CT (HRCT). (**A**) Seven-mm section acquired helically shows a unilateral reticulonodular infiltrate in the right upper lobe. (**B**) One-mm axial HRCT section at the same level as in **A** shows to better advantage findings characteristic of lymphangitic carcinomatosis. In particular, note the clearer depiction of thickened interlobular septa posteriorly, due to dilated lymphatics, resulting in much more easily identifiable polygonal or hexagonal configuration.

Helical (Spiral) Computed Tomography,
edited by Paul M. Silverman.
Lippincott–Raven Publishers, Philadelphia © 1998.

4

Protocols for Helical CT of the Abdomen and Pelvis

James A. Brink*, Jay P. Heiken**, and Paul M. Silverman***

*Department of Radiology, Yale University School of Medicine, New Haven,
Connecticut 06510
**Mallinckrodt Institute of Radiology, Washington University School of Medicine,
St. Louis, Missouri 63110
***Division of Abdominal Imaging, Section of Computed Tomography, Georgetown
University Medical Center, Washington, D.C. 20007

Helical CT has improved established abdominal computed tomography (CT) examinations and has created new examinations such as CT colography. Generation of overlapping images from a single x-ray exposure, suppression of motion artifact, and elimination of respiratory misregistration have heightened the elegance of routine abdominal CT examinations. These same technical advantages have also led to the development of new applications. Advanced three-dimensional postprocessing applications permit simulated endoscopy and allow the radiologist to view anatomy from within any lumen or anatomic space within the abdomen, such as within the bladder or colon. Simulated colonoscopy may be performed with perspective volume rendering of closely spaced helical CT images. A single helical CT angiogram may serve as the sole preoperative imaging test for abdominal aortic aneurysms. Thus helical CT is the cornerstone of many advanced abdominal CT applications (1,2).

HELICAL CT SCAN PARAMETERS

The choice of helical CT scanning parameters greatly affects image quality and anatomic fidelity in routine abdominal CT applications as well as such specialized applications as CT colography. Collimation, table feed, reconstruction interval, and scan timing parameters must be selected carefully to achieve satisfactory results. Despite our best efforts, resolution along the longitudinal axis is an order of magnitude worse than transaxial resolution (typically less than 1 mm). Because many helical abdominal CT applications may be improved with longitudinal reformations for understanding complex anatomy, maximizing longitudinal resolution is critical to proper depiction of small structures on coronal or sagittal two- or three-dimensional reformations. Decreasing the collimation, table feed, and reconstruction interval increases longitudinal resolution. However, reduction of each of these parameters results in certain tradeoffs. Pixel noise increases with decreasing collimation. The scan coverage that may be achieved with a given scan duration will be constrained by limiting the table feed to a pitch of 1.0 (pitch = table increment per gantry rotation/collimation). Finally, the degree to which reconstructed images overlap increases as the reconstruction interval is decreased from below the effective slice thickness. This increases processing time, physician review time, and data storage requirements for a given helical CT scan (3,4).

Helical CT applications requiring high detail such as quantifying renal arterial stenoses mandates that thin collimation settings (1–2 mm) are used. However, x-ray tube output limitations often result in unacceptable levels of pixel noise, especially in abdominal and pelvic imaging in obese patients. Consequently, such applications are performed with 3–5-mm collimation. One should choose the lowest collimation setting possible to maximize longitudinal resolution as long as pixel noise is not prohibitive. Scan coverage will be limited if the table feed is held to a pitch of 1.0. Although increasing the pitch will decrease longitudinal resolution by broadening the section sensitivity profile, the penalty is not as severe as if a higher collimation setting were chosen solely to permit performance of the scan with a lower pitch setting. Increasing the pitch up to 2.0 may permit the choice of a lower collimation setting without compromising scan coverage. Here, choice of a lower collimation and higher pitch improves longitudinal resolution relative to choice of a higher collimation and lower pitch settings (3).

Consider an ideal helical CT scanner with integer-selectable collimation settings, including 4-mm and 5-mm settings. If a volume 10 cm in length must be scanned in a 20-sec breath-hold, 5 mm/sec table feed must be used (presuming a 1-sec gantry rotation). If pixel noise is not prohibitive with the lower collimation setting, the 4-mm collimation setting (pitch = 1.25) should be selected instead of the 5-mm setting (pitch = 1.0), since the section sensitivity profile is narrower with the 4-mm setting (Full Width at Half Maximum (FWHM) = 4.3 versus 5.0 mm) (4).

Selection of the lower collimation setting must be appropriate for the patient's body habitus and the organ of interest. A minimum collimation setting of 3 mm should be used for abdominal or pelvic imaging in an obese individual because of the severity of image noise associated with lower collimation settings. Although one might suspect that increasing the pitch increases image noise (for a given collimation setting), theoretical predictions indicate that image noise is independent of pitch and is proportional to kilovoltage, tube current, and collimation (5).

Although increasing pitch does not affect image noise and only minimally broadens the effective slice thickness, choice of a low-collimation, high-pitch combination worsens low-contrast detectability. This is because choice of a lower collimation setting will increase image noise, which reduces low-contrast detectability. In addition, broadening of the section-sensitivity profile (which describes the slice thickness) also results in lower image contrast. Thus choice of a low-collimation, high-pitch combination is appropriate for high-contrast imaging problems such as CT angiography and thoracic imaging. It is less appropriate for low-contrast imaging problems such as routine abdominal or hepatic imaging.

Increasing the pitch will also enhance interpolation artifacts in addition to decreasing low-contrast detectability. The stair-step artifact is one such artifact observed along high-contrast interfaces oriented oblique to the direction of patient travel (6,7). For example, in CT angiography of the abdominal aorta, these are seen as regular discontinuities along the common iliac arteries. Although the artifacts are not created by increasing the pitch, they become more conspicuous with increasing pitch because they are more widely spaced. The subtle change in these artifacts imposed by increasing pitch from 1 to 2 are not substantial and do not significantly compromise the quality of most three-dimensional imaging applications. However, manufacturers tell us that interpolation artifacts become too severe if the pitch is increased above 2. Thus for most clinical applications the upper limit should be a pitch of 2.

The retrospective review of helical CT data increases longitudinal resolution, permitting generation of highly overlapping images from a single x-ray exposure even though simultaneous movement of the table during gantry rotation results in slight broadening of the section sensitivity profile and a decrease in longitudinal resolution. Of these two competing effects, the increase in longitudinal resolution due to image overlap predominates so long as modern 180-degree interpolation algorithms are used. Choice of the reconstruction interval is a compromise between such practical considerations as image processing time, physician review time, data storage requirements, and the maximal longitudinal resolution that one may achieve with highly overlapping images. The benefits of producing images that overlap by 50% have been shown in phantom and clinical studies (8,9). However, higher degrees of overlap do not result in additional benefit because the relationship between longitudinal resolution and image overlap is not linear at higher levels of overlap. Investigators agree that at least 50% overlap should be used in most CT applications (10,11).

LIVER

Hepatic CT requires 1.5–2.5 min to image the entire liver with conventional incremental CT technique. Consequently, the entire liver is generally not imaged with conventional CT during the optimum postenhancement liver scanning interval (i.e., the time after achievement of high hepatic enhancement levels but prior to the onset of equilibrium) (12,13). The relatively short scanning time of helical CT overcomes this problem because the entire liver can be imaged during the peak of hepatic enhancement without scanning during the equilibrium phase. Because a helical CT scan is completed within a very short scanning interval (i.e., 30–40 sec), a uniphasic injection using a relatively rapid flow rate (e.g., 3 mL/sec) is most advantageous (14,15). For helical CT of the liver, it is generally necessary to use a longer scan delay than is used for conventional CT. However, the optimal scan delay depends on the volume of contrast material and the rate at which it is injected. For most IV contrast injection protocols, a scan delay of 60–80 sec is appropriate. At very rapid rates, such as 5 mL/sec, a delay of 50 sec may be employed. Table 1 lists recommended scan delays for various IV contrast material injection protocols.

TABLE 1. *Recommended scan delays for lepatic helical CT*

Volume (mL)	Injection rate (mL/sec)	Delay (sec)
100	1.5	70
100	2	60
100	3	55
125	1.5	85
125	2	70
125	3	60
150	1.5	100
150	2	85
150	3	70
150	4	55
150	5	50
200	1.5	135
200	2	110
200	3	85
200	4	70
200	5	60

Note: Power injection of central lines and port-a-catheters should be performed at 1.5 mL/sec. The attending radiologist should review the topogram or a recent chest x-ray to be sure that the line is in good position. Central venous catheters placed via a peripheral vein should not be power injected. Hand injection is acceptable for these catheters.

In recent years, semi-automated techniques have emerged to determine the adequacy of contrast enhancement during infusion of contrast material intended for a diagnostic scan (i.e., computer automated scan technology [CAST] or bolus tracking). Such techniques generally acquire a series of low x-ray dose transaxial images at a predetermined level that is representative of the scan volume (16,17). Once contrast enhancement is deemed adequate (by the operator or by the computer), acquisition of the low-dose transaxial scans is terminated and the diagnostic scan is commenced at the beginning of the intended scan volume. Data have shown this technique to be highly effective and to achieve better contrast enhancement than with the standard fixed-delay approach. A threshold of 50 HU above baseline for enhancement has been recommended (16).

Because of the speed of helical CT, one may scan the liver during either the hepatic arterial or the portal venous phase of enhancement, or during both phases. As most metastases are hypovascular compared with normal hepatic parenchyma when imaged during the portal venous phase of enhancement, conventional dynamic incremental hepatic CT scanning protocols were designed to optimize imaging during this phase of contrast enhancement. However, many primary hepatic neoplasms and some metastases are iso- or hypervascular and can become isoattenuating during the portal venous enhancement phase. Because of their vascularity, such neoplasms may be better imaged during the arterial phase of hepatic enhancement. However, dynamic incremental scanning requires too much time to image the liver during both the arterial and portal venous enhancement phases. Helical CT provides the potential to image the entire liver twice, once during the arterial and once during the portal venous enhancement phases. The arterial phase scan is usually begun 20 sec after initiation of contrast injection, although one group has reported improved accuracy in the timing of this scan when triggered by a CAST synonymous with the bolus tracking approach (18). Such dual-phase or biphasic hepatic imaging is used in selected patients who are at high risk for vascular hepatic neoplasms. Recent studies of patients with hepatocellular carcinoma and various types of hypervascular metastases have demonstrated an 8% to 13% increase in lesion detection with dual-phase helical CT compared with portal venous phase imaging alone (19–22). In comparisons of dual-phase CT and dynamic MR imaging, arterial phase MR imaging has been shown to be slightly superior for hepatic lesion detection (23,24). However, for delayed phase imaging (greater than 180 sec), helical CT was significantly better than MR imaging (24). Hepatic lesion characterization may also be improved by imaging during the arterial, portal, and equilibrium phases of contrast enhancement (25).

The continuous data acquisition of helical CT offers additional advantages for hepatic imaging as compared with standard incremental scanning. These include the potential for improved lesion detection due to elimination of respiratory misregistration and retrospective image reconstruction at arbitrary positions along the z-axis and the production of high-quality multiplanar images. Helical CT with smaller interscan spacing increases confidence in detection and the overall detection rate of focal liver lesions. By viewing images of the liver reconstructed at 4-mm intervals (8-mm collimation, 50% overlap), 7% more lesions could be detected in a group of patients with liver metastases, as compared with viewing contiguous images of the same patients reconstructed at 8-mm intervals (9). Three-dimensional size measurements of liver metastases in patients undergoing cancer treatment have been found to be reproducible with helical CT images acquired in a breath-hold and reconstructed with 25% overlap (26). Multiplanar and three-dimensional reconstructions of the volume-acquired data can be useful in precisely localizing and defining the extent of hepatic tumors prior to resection. These advantages make helical CT the preferred method of performing CT arterial portography (27,28).

The amount of intravenous contrast material required for hepatic enhancement may be reduced with helical CT. Adequate hepatic enhancement has been reported with an iodine dose that is 25% lower than that with conventional CT (15). In thin patients, the potential to reduce contrast dose is even more pronounced and a reduction of up to 40% is possible. Contrast material reduction is possible when helical scan technology is coupled with CAST as a means of determining enhancement adequacy (29).

PANCREAS

With helical CT, high levels of pancreatic enhancement may be achieved that help accentuate the difference between normal pancreas and tumor, permitting exquisite definition of arterial and venous involvement by pancreatic disease (30,31). Pancreatic enhancement during the early phase (20–40-sec delay) of dual-phase helical CT often is significantly greater than that seen using a standard delay (50–70 sec) (32,33). In addition, smaller amounts of contrast material may produce equivalent or superior peripancreatic vascular opacification as compared with standard CT (31). The ability to scan the entire pancreas during arterial enhancement and to reconstruct images at overlapping intervals may improve the ability of CT to demonstrate and stage small pancreatic adenocarcinomas, although this potential benefit of helical CT has yet to be demonstrated in a prospective study (34). Three-dimensional rendering using maximum intensity projection (MIP), shaded surface display (SSD), or volume rendering (VRT) may be useful in confirming vascular encasement or invasion.

Because islet cell tumors are typically hypervascular, they should be more conspicuous during the early phase of dual-phase pancreatic helical CT. Although this phenomenon has been described anecdotally (30,35), a large prospective study confirming this finding has not emerged. Instead, a small series of 10 patients with 11 surgically proved islet cell tumors was published recently in which dual-phase helical CT was performed with 5-mm slice thickness (36). All tumors larger than 5 mm and one of three lesions less than 5 mm in diameter were detected with dual-phase pancreatic helical CT. Two lesions were better seen during the arterial phase, and two lesions were better seen on the parenchymal phase images. Thus the arterial and parenchymal phases may be complementary, and both phases may be necessary to fully evaluate patients with suspected islet cell tumors.

BILIARY TREE AND PORTA HEPATIS

The porta hepatis may be difficult to evaluate with standard CT because of its complicated anatomy and oblique orientation. With helical CT images reconstructed with at least 50% overlap, the radiologist may perform longitudinal reformations of the porta hepatis in any plane to optimally depict important vascular and biliary structures contained within. Detection of common bile duct stones and strictures may be improved with contrast-enhanced helical CT, particularly when an interactive cine display console is used to determine the most beneficial planes for displaying the biliary tree (37).

Three-dimensional cholangiographic quality images may be produced following intravenous infusion of a biliary contrast agent (38–41). However, one must accept the toxicity associated with use of an intravenous biliary agent when considering use of this technique. In addition, excretion of these biliary agents is decreased in the setting of biliary obstruction. Thus successful depiction of the biliary tree is impeded in the very population in whom it is most desirable. However, two-dimensional reformations of the bile duct may be generated from routine helical scans performed with intravenous contrast material (42). Such images depict the bile duct with negative contrast as a low-attenuation structure against background tissue enhanced with intravenous contrast material. Such images may be helpful in depicting complex anatomy in the hepatoduodenal ligament, especially in the setting of invasive gall-bladder or pancreatic cancer.

KIDNEY

Small renal masses that are indeterminate by other imaging techniques may be better evaluated with helical CT (43,44). As in the liver and pancreas, the lack of respiratory misregistration artifacts and the ability to reconstruct images at overlapping intervals make it less likely that a small mass will be missed.

With helical renal CT, the kidneys may be imaged during four distinct phases of contrast enhancement: the precontrast phase, the corticomedullary phase, the nephrographic phase, and the excretory phase. The corticomedullary phase occurs between 30 and 60 sec, and the nephrographic phase occurs between 100 and 130 sec following initiation of contrast infusion. Although little has been published regarding characterization of known lesions during these phases, one study has shown greater enhancement of renal neoplasms during the nephrographic phase (45), and another has shown limited detection of renal lesions when imaged only during the corticomedullary phase (46). Of 417 lesions detected in 33 patients, 62% were depicted during the corticomedullary phase, whereas 93% were seen on the nephrographic phase images. When the nephrographic phase images were added to the corticomedullary phase images, the number of medullary lesions detected increased by a factor of 4.4, whereas the number of cortical lesions increased by a factor of 1.2.

A recent study by Szolar and colleagues evaluated the use of multiphasic helical CT for the detection and characterization of small (<3 cm) renal masses (47). As suggested in prior studies, the authors found that nephrographic phase scans enabled greater lesion detection and better characterization of small renal masses than corticomedullary phase scans. However, there are several theoretical advantages of scanning during the corticomedullary phase that mitigate against discarding it entirely. Tumor vascularity may be better appreciated during the corticomedullary phase (48). Corticomedullary differentiation can be helpful in distinguishing normal variants such as prominent columns of Bertin or dromedary humps from renal masses (45). Subtle asymmetries in the cortical nephrogram that result from renal artery stenosis or ureteral obstruction may be more apparent during the nephrographic phase than during the corticomedullary phase. Thus the cost versus benefit of multiphasic helical renal CT must be elicited in future studies, especially with regard to these theoretical advantages of imaging during the corticomedullary phase of enhancement.

Two- and three-dimensional reformations may be helpful in defining certain types of renal abnormalities. Three-dimensional reconstructions may provide useful information in the staging of renal cell carcinoma and in planning renal-sparing surgery in selected patients (49). Multiplanar reformations of dynamic arterial and venous phase helical CT images in patients with ureteropelvic junction (UPJ) obstruction help identify large crossing vessels at the UPJ prior to endopyelotomy (50). Transaxial renal helical CT images, in combination with three-dimensional reconstructions, have been shown to be suitable replacements for intravenous urography and angiography in the assessment of living renal donors (51). Finally, unenhanced transaxial helical CT images, in combination with two-dimensional reformations, have been shown to be feasible replacements for intravenous urography in the assessment of patients with acute flank pain (52,53).

Helical CT performed without intravenous contrast material may substitute for intravenous urography in patients with acute flank pain. Direct visualization of renal or ureteral calculi, and secondary signs of stone disease—including hydronephrosis, hydroureter, and perinephric/periureteral soft-tissue infiltration—may be seen in patients with acute renal colic (54). In addition, extraurinary causes of acute flank pain may be revealed when urinary calculi are not responsible for the patient's symptoms. Although the x-ray dose associated with the helical CT examination is greater than that with a tailored intravenous urogram, the helical CT examination is performed much more quickly and does not require intravenous contrast material.

COMPLEX ANATOMIC RELATIONSHIPS/CT COLOGRAPHY

Interpretative difficulties arising from complex anatomic relationships may be clarified with multiplanar reformations of helical CT images. Images targeted to the area of concern that overlap by at least 50% may be reconstructed retrospectively from the raw projection data. Multiplanar images reconstructed from these images may be useful, for example, in determining the site of origin of large abdominal masses or in localizing peridiaphragmatic abnormalities to the abdomen, diaphragm, or thorax (55).

Recently, investigators have proposed using helical CT of the colon to detect colonic polyps (56,57). However, the technique is still in its infancy. Some advocate use of two-dimensional reformations to ''straighten'' the colon, whereas others suggest performing three-dimensional perspective volume or surface rendering to fly through the colon simulating colonoscopy.

GENERAL COMMENTS

1. For helical CT examinations of the abdomen, respiration should be suspended. Prolonged breath-holding can be facilitated by hyperventilating the patient with three or four deep breaths in rapid succession just before beginning the helical CT scan.
2. In general, use a pitch of 1.0–1.5 (i.e., table increment equal to or 50% greater than collimation). In some cases it will be necessary to use a pitch of 2.0 to cover the entire volume of interest.
3. Bolus tracking (CAST) may be used to determine the delay time for initiation of hepatic imaging. Position three regions of interest (ROIs) in the liver parenchyma. Initiate scanning when at least two of the three ROIs reach 50 HU of enhancement.
4. Bolus tracking should not to be used in dual-phase helical CT examinations of the liver or pancreas, or in CT angiography applications.
5. Field of view (FOV): Most abdominal examinations should be reconstructed with a FOV targeted to the abdominal wall except for patients with a history of melanoma or other significant abnormalities in the subcutaneous tissues. For these cases, the FOV should be increased to include the entire abdominal circumference. In extremely large patients, a second image reconstruction targeted to the abdominal wall may be required. In these instances, re-review of the helical CT data may be performed retrospectively. Some specialized protocols may call for a FOV targeted to the structure of interest such as the kidney or aorta.
6. Oral contrast material: Abdominal and abdominal/pelvic CT patients are given 600–800 mL of oral contrast material to drink 45–60 min prior to their examination, and an additional 200 mL just prior to scanning. Either water-soluble contrast solutions or barium

solutions may be used, depending on the clinical indication for the examination as well as several technical and environmental factors. Dilute water-soluble contrast may be preferred for outpatients to increase bowel motility and promote uniform bowel opacification. Water-soluble contrast material is also given to postoperative/posttraumatic patients in whom bowel perforation or leakage is a possibility. Dilute barium may be preferred for routine inpatients, largely because of ease of contrast delivery to the patient floors, and to avoid the increase in bowel motility associated with water soluble agents.

Regardless of the initial oral contrast material chosen, patients may be given a large cup of water to ingest immediately before their abdominal CT scan. This is better tolerated by the patients than another cup of contrast material and may provide better definition of the gastric wall, especially if IV contrast material has been administered.

REFERENCES

1. Brink JA. Spiral CT angiography of the abdomen and pelvis: interventional applications. *Abdom Imaging* 1997; 22:365–372.
2. Brink JA, McFarland EG, Heiken JP. Helical/spiral computed body tomography. *Clin Rad* 1997;52:489–503.
3. Brink JA. Technical aspects of helical (spiral) CT. *Radiol Clin North Am* 1995;33:825–841.
4. Brink JA, Davros WJ. Helical/spiral CT: technical principles. In: Zeman RK, ed. *Helical/spiral CT: a practical approach.* New York: McGraw-Hill, 1995;1–26.
5. Wang G, Vannier MW. Maximum volume coverage in spiral computed tomography scanning. *Acad Radiol* 1996;3:423–428.
6. Wang G, Vannier MW. Stair-step artifacts in three-dimensional helical CT: an experimental study. *Radiology* 1994;191:79–83.
7. Polacin A, Kalender WA, Brink JA, Vannier MW. Measurement of slice sensitivity profiles in spiral CT. *Med Phys* 1994;21:133–140.
8. Kasales CJ, Hopper KD, Ariola DN, et al. Reconstructed helical CT scans: improvement in *z*-axis resolution compared with overlapped and nonoverlapped conventional CT scans. *AJR* 1995;164:1281–1284.
9. Urban BA, Fishman EK, Kuhlman JE, Kawashima A, Hennessey JG, Siegelman SS. Detection of focal hepatic lesions with spiral CT: comparison of 4- and 8-mm interscan spacing. *AJR* 1993;160:783–785.
10. Wang G, Brink JA, Vannier MW. Theoretical FWTM values in helical CT. *Med Phys* 1994;21:753–754.
11. Kalender WA, Polacin A, Suss C. A comparison of conventional and spiral CT: an experimental study on the detection of spherical lesions. *JCAT* 1994;18:167–176.
12. Foley WD. Dynamic hepatic CT. *Radiology* 1989;170:617–622.
13. Heiken JP, Brink JA, McClennan BL, Sagel SS, Forman HP, DiCroce J. Dynamic contrast-enhanced CT of the liver: comparison of contrast medium injection rates and uniphasic and biphasic injection protocols. *Radiology* 1993;187:327–331.
14. Foley WD, Hoffmann RG, Quiroz FA, Kahn CE, Perret RS. Hepatic helical CT: contrast material injection protocol. *Radiology* 1994;192:367–371.
15. Brink JA, Heiken JP, Forman HP, Sagel SS, Molina PL, Brown PC. Hepatic spiral CT: reduction of dose of intravenous contrast material. *Radiology* 1995;197:83–88.
16. Silverman PM, Roberts S, Tefft MC, et al. Helical CT of the liver: clinical application of an automated computer technique, SmartPrep, for obtaining images with optimal contrast enhancement. *AJR* 1995;165:73–78.
17. Kopka L, Funke M, Fischer U, Vosshenrich R, Oestmann JW, Grabbe E. Parenchymal liver enhancement with bolus-triggered helical CT: preliminary clinical results. *Radiology* 1995;195:282–284.
18. Kopka L, Rodenwaldt J, Fischer U, Mueller DW, Oestmann JW, Grabbe E. Dual-phase helical CT of the liver: effects of bolus tracking and different volumes of contrast material. *Radiology* 1996;201:321–326.
19. Oliver III JH, Baron RL, Federle MP, Rockette Jr HE. Detecting hepatocellular carcinoma: value of unenhanced or arterial phase CT imaging or both used in conjunction with conventional portal venous phase contrast-enhanced CT imaging. *AJR* 1996;167:71–77.
20. Baron RL, Oliver III JH, Dodd III GD, Nalesnik M, Holbert BL, Carr B. Hepatocellular carcinoma: evaluation with biphasic, contrast-enhanced, helical CT. *Radiology* 1996;199:505–511.
21. Hollett MD, Jeffrey RB, Nino-Murcia M, Jorgensen MJ, Harris DP. Dual-phase helical CT of the liver: value of arterial phase scans in the detection of small malignant hepatic neoplasms. *AJR* 1995;164:879–884.
22. Bonaldi VM, Bret PM, Reinhold C, Atri M. Helical CT of the liver: value of an early hepatic arterial phase. *Radiology* 1995;197:357–363.
23. Oi H, Murakami R, Kim T, Matsushita M, Kishimoto H, Nakamura H. Dynamic MR imaging and early-phase helical CT for detecting small intrahepatic metastases of hepatocellular carcinoma. *AJR* 1996;166:369–374.
24. Yamashita YY, Mitsuzaki KM, Yi T, et al. Small hepatocellular carcinoma in patients with chronic liver damage: prospective comparison of detection with dynamic MR imaging and helical CT of the whole liver. *Radiology* 1996;200:79–84.

25. Van Leeuwen MS, Noordzij J, Feldberg MAM, Hennipman AH, Doornewaard H. Focal liver lesions: characterization with triphasic spiral CT. *Radiology* 1996;201:327–336.
26. Van Hoe L, Van Cutsem E, Vergote I, et al. Size quantification of liver metastases in patients undergoing cancer treatment: reproducibility of one-, two-, and three-dimensional measurements determined with spiral CT. *Radiology* 1997;202:671–675.
27. Bluemke DA, Fishman EK. Spiral CT arterial portography of the liver. *Radiology* 1993;186:576–579.
28. Ichikawa T, Ohtomo K, Takhashi S. Hepatocellular carcinoma: detection with double-phase helical CT during arterial portography. *Radiology* 1996;198:284–287.
29. Silverman PM, Roberts SC, Ducic I, et al. Assessment of a technology that permits individualized scan delays on helical hepatic CT: a technique to improve efficiency in use of contrast material. *AJR* 1996;167:79–84.
30. Fishman EK, Wyatt SH, Ney DR, Kuhlman JE, Siegelman SS. Spiral CT of the pancreas with multiplanar display. *AJR* 1992;159:1209–1215.
31. Dupuy DE, Costello P, Ecker CP. Spiral CT of the pancreas. *Radiology* 1992;183:815–818.
32. Lu DSK, Vedantham S, Krasny RM, Kadell B, Berger WL, Reber HA. Two-phase helical CT for pancreatic tumors: pancreatic versus hepatic phase enhancement of tumor, pancreas, and vascular structures. *Radiology* 1996;199:697–701.
33. Hollett MD, Jorgensen MJ, Jeffrey RB. Quantitative evaluation of pancreatic enhancement during dual-phase helical CT. *Radiology* 1995;195:359–361.
34. Bluemke DA, Cameron JL, Hruban RH, et al. Potentially resectable pancreatic adenocarcinoma: spiral CT assessment with surgical and pathologic correlation. *Radiology* 1995;197:381–385.
35. Foley WD. Helical CT: clinical performance and imaging strategies. *Radiographics* 1994;14:894–904.
36. Van Hoe L, Gryspeerdt S, Marchal G, Baert AL, Mertens L. Helical CT for the preoperative localization of islet cell tumors of the pancreas: value of arterial and parenchymal phase images. *AJR* 1995;165:1437–1439.
37. Brink JA, Heiken JP, Balfe DM. Noninvasive cholangiography with spiral CT. *Radiology* 1992;185:141.
38. Van Beers BE, Lacrosse M, Trigaux JP, de Canniere L, De Ronde T, Pringot J. Noninvasive imaging of the biliary tree before or after laparoscopic cholecystectomy: use of three-dimensional spiral CT cholangiography. *AJR* 1994;162:1331–1335.
39. Fleischmann D, Ringl H, Schofl R, et al. Three-dimensional spiral CT cholangiography in patients with suspected obstructive biliary disease: comparison with endoscopic retrograde cholangiography. *Radiology* 1996;198:861–868.
40. Klein HM, Wein B, Truong S, Pfingsten FP, Gunther RW. Computed tomographic cholangiography using spiral scanning and 3D image processing. *Br J Radiol* 1993;66:762–767.
41. Stockberger SM, Wass JL, Sherman S, Lehman GA, Kopecky KK. Intravenous cholangiography with helical CT: comparison with endoscopic retrograde cholangiography. *Radiology* 1994;192:675–680.
42. Heiken JP, Brink JA, Sagel SS. Helical CT: abdominal applications. *Radiographics* 1994;14:919–924.
43. Silverman SG, Seltzer SE, Adams DF, Tumeh SS, Allegra DP, Mellins HZ. Spiral CT of the small indeterminate renal mass: results in 48 patients. *Radiology* 1991;181:125.
44. Silverman SG, Lee BY, Seltzer SE, Bloom DA, Corless CL, Adams DF. Small (≤3 cm) renal masses: correlation of spiral CT features and pathologic findings. *AJR* 1994;163:597–605.
45. Birnbaum BA, Jacobs JE, Ramchandani P. Multiphasic renal CT: comparison of renal mass enhancement during the corticomedullary and nephrographic phases. *Radiology* 1996;200:753–758.
46. Cohan RH, Sherman LS, Korobkin M, Bass JC, Francis IR. Renal masses: assessment of corticomedullary-phase and nephrographic-phase CT scans. *Radiology* 1995;196:445–451.
47. Szolar DH, Kammerhuber F, Altziebler S, et al. Multiphasic helical CT of the kidney: increased conspicuity for detection and characterization of small (<3-cm) renal masses. *Radiology* 1997;202:211–217.
48. Urban BA. The small renal mass: what is the role of multiphasic helical scanning? *Radiology* 1997;202:22–23.
49. Chernoff DM, Silverman SG, Kikinis R, et al. Three-dimensional imaging and display of renal tumors using spiral CT: a potential aid to partial nephrectomy. *Urology* 1994;43:125–129.
50. Quillin SP, Brink JA, Heiken JP, Siegel CL, McClennan BL, Clayman RV. Spiral CT angiography: identification of crossing vessels at the ureteropelvic junction. *AJR* 1996;166:1125–1130.
51. Platt JR, Ellis JH, Korobkin M, Reige KA, Konnak JW, Leichtman AB. Potential renal donors: comparison of conventional imaging with helical CT. *Radiology* 1996;198:419–423.
52. Sommer FG, Jeffrey RBJ, Rubin GD, et al. Detection of ureteral calculi in patients with suspected renal colic: value of reformatted noncontrast helical CT. *AJR* 1995;165:509–513.
53. Smith RC, Verga M, McCarthy S, Rosenfield AT. Diagnosis of acute flank pain: value of unenhanced helical CT. *AJR* 1996;166:97–101.
54. Katz DS, Lane MJ, Sommer FG. Unenhanced helical CT of ureteral stones: incidence of associated urinary tract findings. *AJR* 1996;166:1319–1322.
55. Brink JA, Heiken JP, Semenkovich J, Teefey SA, McClennan BL, Sagel SS. Abnormalities of the diaphragm and adjacent structures: findings on multiplanar spiral CT scans. *AJR* 1994;163:307–310.
56. Rubin GD, Beaulieu CF, Argiro V, et al. Perspective volume rendering of CT and MR images: applications for endoscopic imaging. *Radiology* 1996;199:321–330.
57. Hara AK, Johnson CD, Reed JE, Ehman RL, Ilstrup DM. Colorectal polyp detection with CT colography: two- versus three-dimensional techniques. *Radiology* 1996;200:49–54.

Protocol 1:
ABDOMEN SURVEY (Fig. 1)

INDICATION: *Screening, R/O metastases, evaluate liver*

SCANNER SETTINGS: kVp: 120–140
                             mAs: 210–330

ORAL CONTRAST: 600–800 mL, 45–60 min prior to study initiation.
                             An additional 200 mL given just prior to
                             scanning.

PHASE OF RESPIRATION: Suspended expiration, following hyperventilation

SLICE THICKNESS: 5–8 mm

PITCH: 1.6

HELICAL EXPOSURE TIME: 24–32 sec, remainder scans cluster or single
                             slice

SUPERIOR EXTENT: Dome of the diaphragm

INFERIOR EXTENT: Iliac crest

IV CONTRAST:

Concentration:	LOCM 300–320 mg iodine/mL or HOCM 282 mg iodine/mL (60% solution)
Rate:	2–3 mL/sec
Scan Delay:	70 sec
Total Volume:	125–150 mL

COMMENTS:

1. For three-dimensional imaging, save the raw data, retrospectively reconstruct images at 3–4-mm intervals for three-dimensional model. Keep the series in exact order by location. Do not alter field of view, matrix size, or center within the series.
2. If there is any question of renal abnormalities, rescan the kidneys following medullary and collecting system opacification. These recuts may be done as conventional, cluster, or helical scans. If densely enhancing abnormalities are seen that need to be

differentiated from calcifications, perform a few delayed cuts.

3. Length of coverage can be increased by increasing the pitch beyond 1.6 up to 2.0.

4. The use of overlapping images, 4-mm interscan spacing has been shown to increase lesion detection.

5. If available, a computer automated scan technology (CAST) can be used to scan the liver. A threshold of 50 HU of enhancement over baseline is recommended. Using the full-contrast dose (150 mL), this provides improved contrast enhancement and less interpatient variability. If desired, results equivalent to using 150 mL with a standard fixed delay can be achieved with 125 mL and CAST.

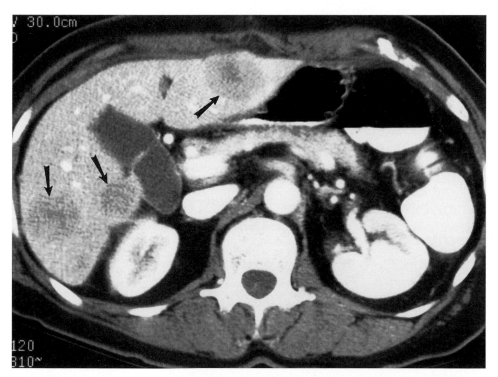

FIG. 1. CT scan at the level of the liver demonstrating excellent vascular and hepatic parenchymal enhancement. Note multiple liver metastases in both lobes (arrows).

Protocol 2:
ABDOMEN AND PELVIS SURVEY (Fig. 2)

INDICATION:	*Tumor staging, abscess*
SCANNER SETTINGS:	kVp: 120–140 mAs: 210–330
ORAL CONTRAST:	600–800 mL, 45–60 min prior to study initiation. An additional 200 mL given just prior to scanning.
PHASE OF RESPIRATION:	Suspended expiration
SLICE THICKNESS:	5–8 mm in abdomen, 7–10 mm in pelvis
PITCH:	1.0–1.6

HELICAL EXPOSURE TIME:	Single Helical Scan: 24–32 sec
	Multiple Helical Scans:
	  First scan duration: 15–20 sec
	  Breathing interval: 10 sec
	  Second scan duration: 15–20 sec

RECONSTRUCTION INTERVAL:	7–8 mm in abdomen; 7–10 mm in pelvis
SUPERIOR EXTENT:	Dome of the diaphragm
INFERIOR EXTENT:	Symphysis pubis

IV CONTRAST:

Concentration:	LOCM 300–320 mg iodine/mL or HOCM 282 mg iodine/mL (60% solution)
Scan Delay:	70 sec
Technique:	Uniphasic or biphasic
Uniphasic:	Rate: 2–3 mL/sec Volume: 125–150 mL

COMMENTS:

1. A uniphasic injection for helical CT is recommended. However, a biphasic injection can be used to slightly prolong the contrast bolus. In very thin (e.g., less than 120 lb) patients it may be possible to use lower mAs for the helical scan. This may allow you to do a longer helix or multiple helices down through the pelvis. Frequently, when the pelvis is scanned, the bladder has not opacified with contrast material. If this is the case, additional 10-mm scans through the bladder may be performed.

2. It is preferable to utilize 330 mAs for patients up to 250 lb and higher, up to 400 mAs in patients over 250 lb.

3. Length of coverage can be increased by increasing the pitch up to 2.0.

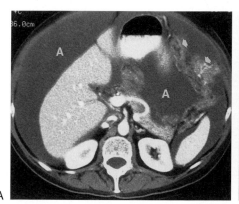 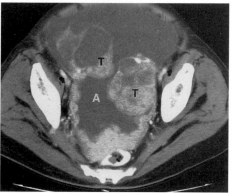

FIG. 2. (**A**) Scan at liver. Note excellent vascular enhancement. Metastases along gastro-splenic ligament identified by soft tissue within fatty ligament (*arrowhead*). Ascites (A). (**B**) Bilateral ovarian carcinomas (T) in pelvis. Excellent vascular enhancement of iliac vessels (*arrowheads*) despite already scanning entire abdomen. Ascites (A).

Protocol 3:
SURVEY FOR ABDOMINAL/PELVIC TRAUMA (Fig. 3)

INDICATION:	*Assess extent of trauma*
SCANNER SETTINGS:	kVp: 120–140 mAs: 210–330
ORAL CONTRAST:	600–800 ml, 45–60 minutes prior to the study initiation or as soon as possible prior to the examination. An additional 200 ml given just prior to scanning.
PHASE OF RESPIRATION:	Suspended expiration
SLICE THICKNESS:	5–8 mm
PITCH:	1.0 or up to 1.6
HELICAL EXPOSURE TIME:	24–32 sec
RECONSTRUCTION INTERVAL:	7–8 mm
SUPERIOR EXTENT:	Dome of the diaphragm
INFERIOR EXTENT:	Symphysis pubis

IV CONTRAST:

Concentration:	LOCM 300–320 mg iodine/mL or HOCM 282 mg iodine/mL (60% solution)
Rate:	2–3 mL/sec
Scan Delay:	60–70 sec
Total Volume:	125–150 mL

COMMENTS:

1. This technique is essentially an abdominal/pelvic survey. It also can be used as a protocol for abdominal trauma. A few noncontrast scans through the spleen can be obtained to observe for acute hemorrhage appearing as high density.
2. As with conventional CT it is imperative to scan the pelvis. Some patients may have a significant intra-abdominal bleed with minimal blood in the abdomen but extensive blood in the pelvis.
3. Remove all leads and extraneous devices prior to scanning.
4. Length of coverage can be increased by increasing the pitch up to 2.0.

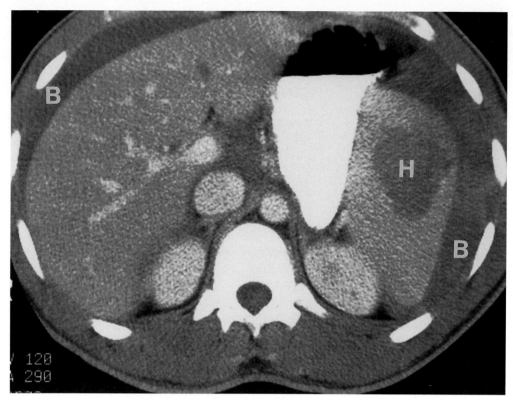

FIG. 3. (**A**) Scan at level of the spleen despite critically ill nature of patient with compromise in cardiac output. A large hematoma (H) is noted in the spleen with surrounding intraperitoneal blood (**B**). The patient received a large volume of fluids for stabilization.

Protocol 4:
THORAX/ABDOMEN (Fig. 4)

INDICATION:	*Combined study; oncologic survey/follow-up*
SCANNER SETTINGS:	kVp: 120–140 mAs: 250–330 (abdomen) 150–250 (thorax)
ORAL CONTRAST:	600–800 mL, 45–60 min prior to study initiation. An additional 200 mL given just prior to scanning.
PHASE OF RESPIRATION:	Suspended inspiration
SLICE THICKNESS:	7–8 mm
PITCH:	1.0–1.6
HELICAL EXPOSURE TIME:	24–32 sec or greater (dependent on technology)
SUPERIOR EXTENT:	Dome of the liver (first series), breath delay (7 sec), and continue to above the aortic arch or if possible to lung apices. Complete thoracic portion and remaining abdominal portion as axial clusters.
INFERIOR EXTENT:	Lower aspect of the liver, scan from caudal to cephalad

IV CONTRAST:

Concentration:	LOCM 300–320 mg iodine/mL or HOCM 282 mg iodine/mL (60 % solution)
Rate:	Technique: Biphasic Phase 1: Rate: 2 mL/sec Volume: 80 mL Phase 2: Rate: 1.5 mL/sec Volume: 70 mL
Scan Delay:	70 sec
Total Volume:	150 mL

SUPERIOR EXTENT: Lung apices helical study, continue inferiorly

INFERIOR EXTENT: Iliac crest

IV CONTRAST:

Concentration:	LOCM 300–320 mg iodine/mL or HOCM 282 mg iodine/mL (60% solution)
Rate:	Technique: Uniphasic Phase 1: Rate: 2-3 mL/sec Volume: 150 mL
Scan Delay:	15–30 sec
Total Volume:	150 mL

COMMENTS:

1. Two different techniques are suggested to study the thorax and abdomen or thorax and abdomen/pelvis. Technique 1 scans the abdomen (liver) first using a cold tube to take maximal advantage of peak mAs for the liver. However, this is less important with modern CT scanners equipped with greater heat capacity x-ray tubes. Technique 2 scans the thorax followed by the abdomen, abdomen/pelvis, and is more simplified, but it does limit the technique through the liver.
2. Length of coverage can be increased by increasing the pitch up to 2.0.

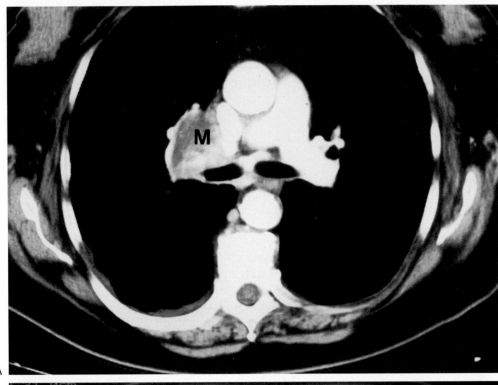

A

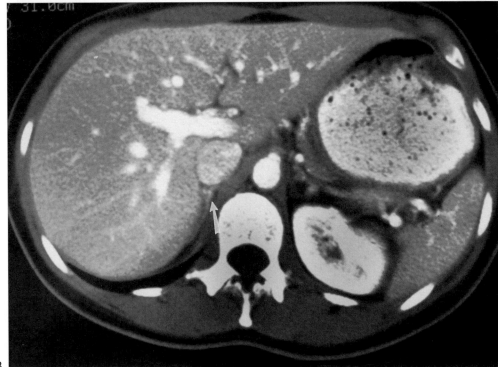

B

FIG. 4. (**A**) CT scan of chest demonstrating large right hilar mass (M). (**B**) Scan at liver and adrenal levels fails to demonstrate adrenal metastases. Normal right adrenal (*arrow*).

Protocol 5:
THORAX/ABDOMEN/PELVIS (Fig. 5)

INDICATION: *Combined study; oncologic screening*

SCANNER SETTINGS: kVp: 120–140
mAs: 210–330 (abdomen portion)
      150–250 (thorax portion)

ORAL CONTRAST: 600–800 mL, 45–60 min prior to study initiation. An additional 200 mL given just prior to scanning.

PHASE OF RESPIRATION: Suspended inspiration

SLICE THICKNESS: 7–8 mm

PITCH: 1.0–1.6

HELICAL EXPOSURE TIME: 24–32 sec or longer if equipment permits

TECHNIQUE 1

SUPERIOR EXTENT: Dome of the liver, (first series), breath delay (7 sec), and continue to above the aortic arch or if possible to lung apices. Complete thoracic portion and remaining pelvic region as axial clusters or individual scans.

INFERIOR EXTENT: Lower aspect of the liver. Scan from caudal to cephalad. Finish at pubic symphysis may do nonhelically.

IV CONTRAST:

Concentration:	LOCM 300–320 mg iodine/mL or HOCM 282 mg iodine/mL (60% solution)
Technique: Biphasic	Phase 1: Rate: 2 mL/sec Volume: 80 mL Phase 2: Rate: 1.5 mL/sec Volume: 70 mL
Scan Delay:	70 sec
Total Volume:	150 mL

TECHNIQUE 2

SUPERIOR EXTENT: Lung apices helical study, continue inferiorly

INFERIOR EXTENT: Pubic symphysis, may do pelvis nonhelically.

IV CONTRAST:

Concentration:	LOCM 300–320 mg iodine/mL or HOCM 282 mg iodine/mL (60% solution)
Scan Delay:	15–30 sec
Total Volume:	150 mL
Technique:	Biphasic
	Phase 1: Rate: 2 mL/sec
	Volume: 80 mL
	Phase 2: Rate: 1.5 mL/sec
	Volume: 70 mL

COMMENTS:

1. Two different techniques are suggested to study the thorax and abdomen or thorax and abdomen/pelvis. Technique 1 scans the abdomen (liver) first using a cold tube to take maximal advantage of peak mAs for the liver. However, this is less important with modern CT scanners equipped with greater heat capacity x-ray tubes. Technique 2 scans the thorax followed by the abdomen, abdomen/pelvis, and is more simplified, but it does limit the technique through the liver.

2. Length of coverage can be increased by increasing the pitch up to 2.0.

3. Scanning of the pelvis may be done nonhelically as needed because of tube-cooling constraints.

→

FIG. 5. (**A**) Excellent control enhancement of mediastinal vasculature. Aorta (A), pulmonary artery (PA). (**B**) CT scan at level of celiac axis (*arrowhead*) and liver demonstrating two hypovascular metastases in the liver (*arrows*). (**C**) Scan at the pelvis shows good pelvic vascular enhancement (*arrows*).

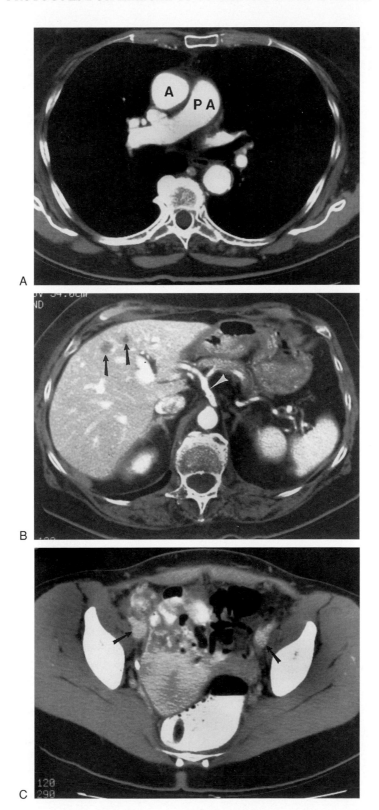

Protocol 6:
PELVIS (Fig. 6)

INDICATION: *Oncologic staging of prostate, cervical, endometrial, or ovarian cancer*

SCANNER SETTINGS: kVp: 120–140
mAs: 165–275

ORAL CONTRAST: Routine, rectal contrast media or air is optional

PHASE OF RESPIRATION: Expiration after routine hyperventiliation

SLICE THICKNESS: 4–5 mm

PITCH: 1.0–1.6

HELICAL EXPOSURE TIME: 24–32 sec

RECONSTRUCTION INTERVAL: 2–3 mm optional for staging pelvic tumors

SUPERIOR EXTENT: Superior iliac crest

INFERIOR EXTENT: Inferior portion of symphysis pubis

IV CONTRAST:

Concentration:	LOCM 300–320 mg iodine/mL or HOCM 282 mg iodine/mL (60% solution)
Rate:	2–3 mL/sec
Scan Delay:	70–80 sec
Total Volume:	100–120 mL

COMMENTS:

1. For pelvic malignancies it is important to begin scanning from the pelvis upward in a caudal–cranial direction. The first scan can be at the level of the lower symphysis pubis. This technique optimizes visualization of pelvic vasculature.
2. Delayed scans can be performed if bladder opacification is desired.
3. Length of coverage can be increased by increasing the pitch up to 2.0.

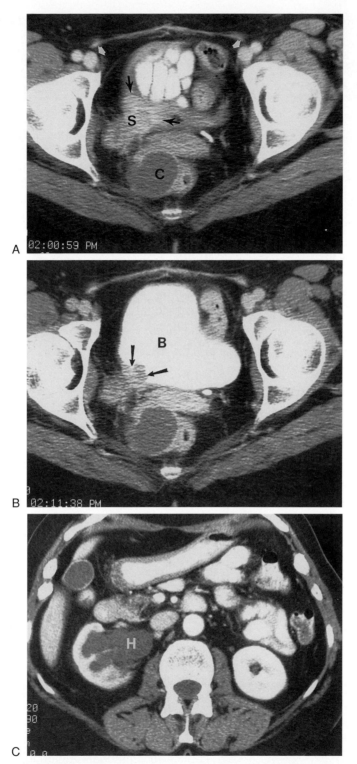

FIG. 6. (**A**) Helical scan of pelvis with excellent vascular enhancement, iliac vessels (*arrowheads*). Note solid (s) and cystic (c) metastases with solid component invading the bladder trigone, causing ureteral obstruction. Enhancement of solid tumor is present during the early phase (*arrows*). (**B**) Delayed scan of pelvis. Bladder is opacified (B). Tumor (*arrows*) invades trigone. (**C**) Scan at level of kidneys showing right hydronephosis (H).

Protocol 7:
DEDICATED LIVER: DUAL PHASE (Fig. 7)

INDICATION: *Primary evaluation of suspected hypervascular hepatic tumors, including focal nodular hyperplasia, hepatic adenoma, hepatocellular carcinoma, hemangioma, and metastases from breast cancer, renal cell carcinoma, islet cell tumors, choriocarcinoma, melanoma, and various sarcomas.*

SCANNER SETTINGS: kVp: 120–140
mAs: 210–330

ORAL CONTRAST: 600–800 mL, 45–60 min prior to study initiation. An additional 200 mL given just prior to scanning.

COLLIMATION: 5 mm for <250 lb, 7–8 mm for ≥250 lb

PITCH: 1.0–1.6

HELICAL EXPOSURE TIME: 24–32 sec

RECONSTRUCTION INTERVAL: 5 mm

SUPERIOR EXTENT: Dome of the diaphragm

INFERIOR EXTENT: Iliac crest

IV CONTRAST:

Concentration:	LOCM 300–350 mg I/mL or HOCM 282 mg I/mL
Rate:	5 mL/sec
Scan Delay:	20 sec for phase 1, 50 sec for phase 2 (or ASAP)
Total Volume:	150 mL

COMMENTS:
1. Unenhanced scans of the liver should be performed prior to contrast injection.
2. If a intrahepatic cholangiocarcinoma is suspected, rescan the liver 15–30 min after bolus.
3. If a hemangioma is suspected, rescan the lesion every 5 min as needed.
4. If the patient's intravenous access catheter cannot accommodate a high injection flow rate, omit arterial phase and perform only venous phase examination. Modify scan delay according to flow rate (Table 1).

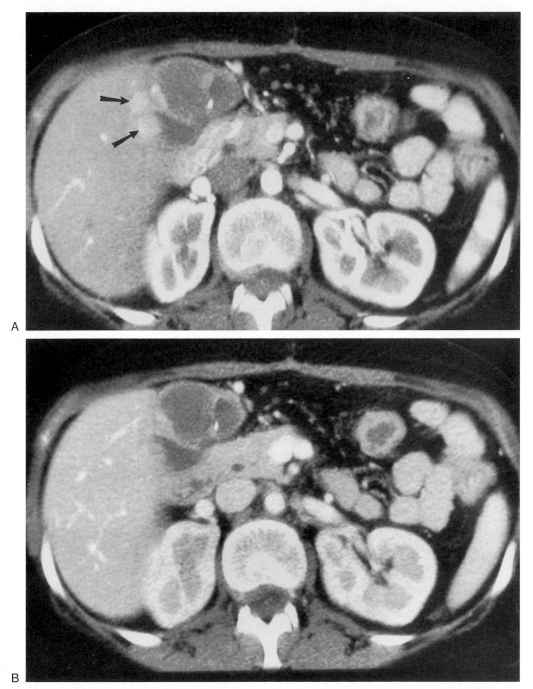

FIG. 7. Hepatocellular carcinoma. (**A**) Arterial phase. (**B**) Portal venous phase. Dual phase helical CT examination reveals better depiction of hyperenhancing tumor nodules (*arrows*) during arterial phase as compared to portal venous phase images. (Reprinted with permission from Brink JA, McFarland EG, Heiken JP. Helical/spiral computed body tomography. *Clin Radiol* 1997;52:489–503.)

Protocol 8:
LIVER: CT ARTERIAL PORTOGRAPHY (CTAP)

INDICATION:	*To determine resectability and to plan surgical resection of neoplastic hepatic disease.*
SCANNER SETTINGS:	kVp: 120–140 mAs: 210–330
ORAL CONTRAST:	None
COLLIMATION:	5 mm for <250 lb, 7–8 mm for ≥250 lb
PITCH:	1.0–1.6
HELICAL EXPOSURE TIME:	24–32 sec
RECONSTRUCTION INTERVAL:	5 mm
SUPERIOR EXTENT:	Dome of the diaphragm
INFERIOR EXTENT:	Iliac crest

IV CONTRAST:

Concentration:	HOCM 200 mg I/mL (or 2:1 dilution of HOCM 282 mg I/mL)
Rate:	2 mL/sec
Scan Delay:	35 sec
Total Volume:	135 mL

COMMENTS:

1. Contrast material is injected via a catheter placed in the superior mesenteric artery.
2. Delayed scans at 4–6 hours may be obtained. After the CTAP has been completed, administer an additional 50 mL of HOCM 282 mg I/mL before the patient leaves the department. Then schedule a repeat CT scan (without additional IV contrast medium) to be done 4–6 hr after the initial scan.

Protocol 9:
PANCREAS (Fig. 8)

INDICATION:	*Evaluate pancreatitis*
SCANNER SETTINGS:	kVp: 120–140 mAs: 210–330
ORAL CONTRAST:	600–800 mL, 45–60 min prior to study initiation. An additional 200 mL given just prior to scanning.
PHASE OF RESPIRATION:	Suspended expiration following hyperventilation
SLICE THICKNESS:	5–8 mm
PITCH:	1.0–1.6
HELICAL EXPOSURE TIME:	24–32 sec
RECONSTRUCTION INTERVAL:	7–8 mm; 4 mm as option
SUPERIOR EXTENT:	Dome of the liver
INFERIOR EXTENT:	Iliac crest or inferiorly to the pelvis, depending on extent of disease.

IV CONTRAST:

Concentration:	LOCM 300–350 mg iodine/mL
Rate:	2–3 mL/sec
Scan Delay:	40–60 sec
Total Volume:	100–150 mL

COMMENTS:

1. This protocol allows scanning from the diaphragm to the iliac crest. This covers the entire area typically involved in pancreatitis. Occasionally, additional scans may be needed if pseudocysts extend upward into the mediastinum or distally into the pelvis.
2. Intravenous contrast media is important to evaluate for viable pancreatic tissue amidst extensive pancreatic inflammatory disease in order to assess for prognostic factors.
3. Length of coverage can be increased by increasing the pitch up to 2.0.
4. Preliminary noncontrast scans of the pancreas are useful to assess for hemorrhagic pancreatitis.

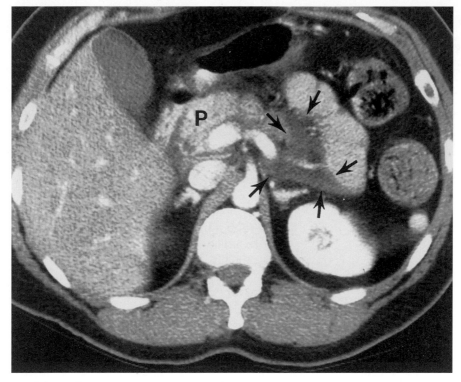

FIG. 8. Scan at level of pancreas (P) showing peripancreatic fluid (*arrows*).

Protocol 10:
DEDICATED PANCREAS: DUAL PHASE
(Figs. 9 and 10)

INDICATION: *Primary evaluation of known or suspected pancreatic neoplasms. Dedicated pancreas study.*

SCANNER SETTINGS: kVp: 120–140
mAs: 210–330

ORAL CONTRAST: 600–800 mL, 45–60 min prior to study initiation. An additional 200 mL given just prior to scanning

COLLIMATION: 3 mm for <250 lb, 5 mm for ≥250 lb

PITCH: 1.0–1.6

HELICAL EXPOSURE TIME: 24–32 sec

**RECONSTRUCTION
  INTERVAL:** 5 mm

SUPERIOR EXTENT: Dome of the diaphragm

INFERIOR EXTENT: Third portion of the duodenum (start)

IV CONTRAST:

Concentration:	LOCM 300–350 mg I/mL or HOCM 282 mg I/mL
Rate:	5 mL/sec
Scan Delay:	30 sec for phase 1, 50 sec for phase 2 (or ASAP)
Total Volume:	150 mL

COMMENTS:

1. Perform unenhanced scan to determine location of third duodenum.
2. Perform helical scan in caudo-cephalad direction beginning at third duodenum or inferior tip of liver, whichever is more caudal.
3. For suspected islet cell tumors, the liver should be scanned during both postcontrast phases, and a scan delay of 20 seconds should be used.
4. If the patient's intravenous access catheter cannot accommodate a high injection flow

rate, omit arterial phase and perform only venous phase examination. Modify scan delay according to flow rate (see Table 1).

5. Water or carbonated beverages may be substituted for positive oral contrast material when three-dimensional images are planned.

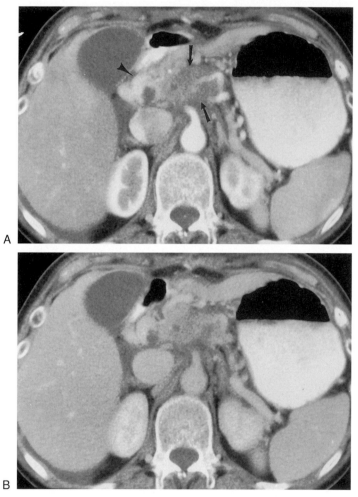

A

B

FIG. 9. Pancreatic adenocarcinoma. (**A**) Arterial phase. (**B**) Portal venous phase. Dual-phase pancreatic helical CT examinations demonstrates better depiction of vascular encasement by hypoenhancing tumor (*arrows*) during the arterial phase than during the portal venous phase. Normally enhancing pancreatic tissue (*arrowhead*) is seen surrounding the dilated common bile duct at this level. (Reprinted with permission from Brink JA, McFarland EG, Heiken JP. Helical/spiral computed body tomography. *Clin Radiol* 1997;52:489–503.)

FIG. 10. Gastrinoma in patient with MEN1. (**A**) Arterial phase. (**B**) Portal venous phase of dual-phase helical pancreatic CT demonstrates a small hyperenhancing nodule (*arrow*) in the pancreatic tail adjacent to a pancreatic cyst to better advantage during the arterial phase than during the portal venous phase. This nodule corresponds to a small gastrinoma which was also identified as a brightly enhancing nodule at digital subtraction angiography (**C**). (Reprinted with permission from Brink JA, McFarland EG, Heiken JP. Helical/spiral computed body tomography. *Clin Radiol* 1997;52:489–503.)

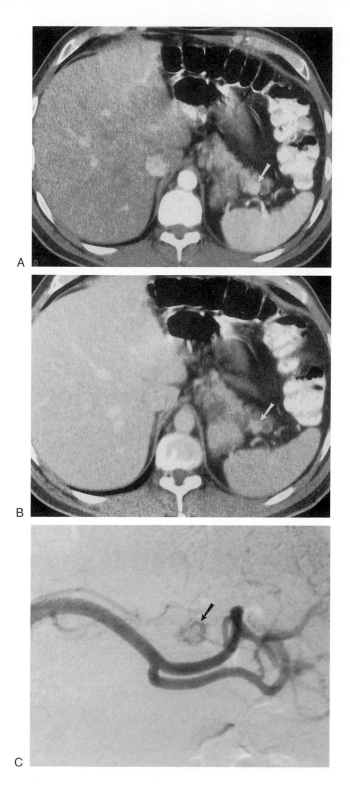

Protocol 11:
SPLEEN SURVEY (Fig. 11)

INDICATION:

SCANNER SETTINGS: kVp: 120
                              mAs: 210–330

ORAL CONTRAST: Optional

PHASE OF RESPIRATION: Expiration after routine hyperventilation

SLICE THICKNESS: 7–8 mm

PITCH: 1.0–1.6

HELICAL EXPOSURE TIME: 24–32 sec

**RECONSTRUCTION
  INTERVAL:**   4–8 mm

SUPERIOR EXTENT: Dome of liver

INFERIOR EXTENT: Superior iliac crest

IV CONTRAST:

Concentration:	LOCM 300–320 mg iodine/mL or HOCM 282 mg iodine/mL (60% solution)
Rate:	2–3 mL/sec
Scan Delay:	60–70 sec
Total Volume:	100 mL-150 mL

COMMENTS:

1. One of the difficulties in evaluating the spleen is that the spleen normally will have a mottled enhancement pattern when contrast is injected dynamically or with spiral CT scanning. Therefore it is best to wait to scan for about 60 sec after contrast injection begins. Occasionally, delayed scans will be needed in equivocal cases. The irregular splenic enhancement is most common in patients with decreased cardiac output.

2. In addition to a mottled appearance the spleen may be striated, or occasionally

confluent curvilinear lucencies may even mimic lesions.
3. Length of coverage can be increased by increasing the pitch up to 2.0.

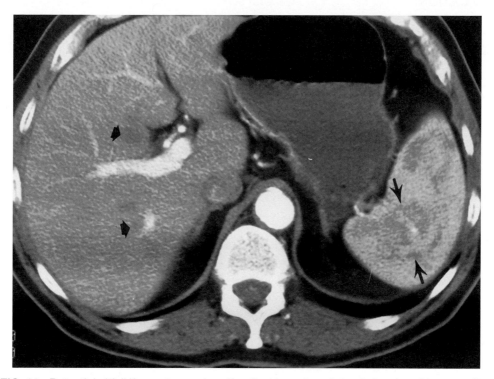

FIG. 11. Potential pitfall if scan too early or if patient has altered circulation time. Note excellent enhancement of aorta and portal vein but unopacified vessels in lever (*arrowheads*). The serpiginous lucencies in the spleen (*arrows*) are a normal variant not be confused with pathology or trauma.

Protocol 12:
KIDNEYS (Fig. 12)

INDICATION:	*General screening abdomen/kidneys, renal vein thrombosis, or other renal abnormalities*
SCANNER SETTINGS:	kVp: 120–140 mAs: 210–330
ORAL CONTRAST:	600–800 mL, 45–60 min prior to study initiation. An additional 200 mL given just prior to scanning.
PHASE OF RESPIRATION:	Suspended expiration
SLICE THICKNESS:	4–8 mm (see comments)
PITCH:	1.0–1.4
HELICAL EXPOSURE TIME:	24–30 sec
RECONSTRUCTION INTERVAL:	5–7 mm, optionally 3–5 mm
SUPERIOR EXTENT:	Above the kidneys (through left adrenal). Initially, noncontrast scans, followed by contrast scans.
INFERIOR EXTENT:	Below the kidneys.
ADDITIONAL SCANS:	Scan entire abdomen as axial clusters or individual scans from just above the dome of the diaphragm to iliac crest at slice thickness of 7–10 mm (see comment 2).

IV CONTRAST:

Concentration:	LOCM 300–320 mg iodine/mL or HOCM 282 mg iodine/mL (60% solution)
Rate:	2–3 mL/sec
Scan Delay:	60–70 sec
Total Volume:	150 mL

COMMENTS:

1. Do not use this protocol for suspected renal artery stenosis. This requires the use of 3-mm slice thickness images.
2. Many institutions and practices perform

noncontrast scans followed by contrast-enhanced scans after a 60–70-sec delay. This results in excellent corticomedullary junctional anatomy images. To avoid missing unopacified medulla, delayed scans are used.

3. Use 5-mm slice thickness if patient is less than 200 lb or the field of view is 37 cm or less. Use 7-mm slice thickness if the patient weighs between 200 and 250 lb or the field of view is 38–40 cm.

4. Do not perform helical scan if patient is more than 250 lb or field of view is above 40 cm.

5. Noncontrast-enhanced scans allow detection of renal calculi.

6. Length of coverage can be increased by increasing the pitch up to 2.0. However, for detection of small renal masses, narrower collimation can be used with increased pitch, or just employ generally narrow collimation 4–6 mm.

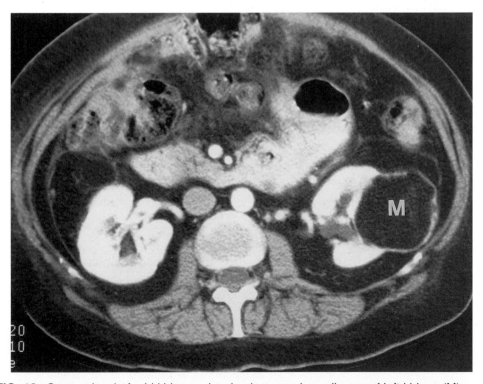

FIG. 12. Scan at level of mid-kidneys showing large angiomyolipoma of left kidney (M).

Protocol 13:
KIDNEYS: DUAL PHASE (Fig. 13)

INDICATION: *Primary evaluation of known or suspected renal neoplasms or other noncalculous focal renal lesions, dedicated renal study.*

SCANNER SETTINGS: kVp: 120–140
mAs: 210–330

ORAL CONTRAST: 600–800 mL, 45–60 min prior to study initiation. An additional 200 mL given just prior to scanning.

COLLIMATION: 3 mm for <250 lb, 5 mm for ≥250 lb

PITCH: 1.0–1.6

HELICAL EXPOSURE TIME: 24–32 sec

**RECONSTRUCTION
INTERVAL:** 3 mm

SUPERIOR EXTENT: Upper pole of kidneys

INFERIOR EXTENT: Lower pole of kidneys

IV CONTRAST:

Concentration:	LOCM 300–350 mg I/mL or HOCM 282 mg I/mL
Rate:	3 mL/sec
Scan Delay:	30 sec for phase 1, 100 sec for phase 2
Total Volume:	100 mL

COMMENTS:
1. Always perform unenhanced scan for baseline attenuation measurements and to detect calcifications.
2. If the patient's intravenous access catheter cannot accommodate a high injection flow rate, omit cortico-medullary phase 1 and perform only nephrographic phase 2 examination.
3. The second scan during the nephrographic phase of enhancement should be performed through the entire abdomen from the diaphragm to the iliac crests.
4. If transitional cell carcinoma (or other uroepithelial abnormality) is suspected, perform excretory phase scan (10-min delay).

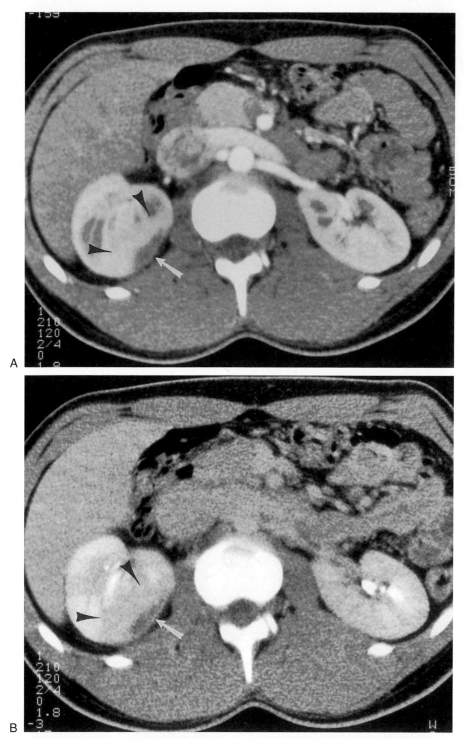

FIG. 13. Page kidney. Corticomedullary phase scan (**A**) reveals a chronic subcapsular hematoma (*arrow*) adjacent to a thickened, enhancing zone of renal cortex (*arrowheads*) that is hypoenhancing on the nephrographic phase scan. (**B**). This is presumed to represent hypervascular, hypofunctioning renal cortex under chronic pressure from the adjacent hematoma. This patient suffered a blow to the right flank 1 year previously and has had uncontrollable hypertension since that time.

Protocol 14:
UPJ OBSTRUCTION (Fig. 14)

INDICATION:	*Evaluation of primary or secondary UPJ obstruction for detection of vessels crossing the UPJ that may be causative or complicate repair.*
SCANNER SETTINGS:	kVp: 120–140 mAs: 210–330
ORAL CONTRAST:	None
PHASE OF RESPIRATION:	Suspended expiration
SLICE THICKNESS:	3 mm for <250 lb, 5 mm for ≥250 lb
PITCH:	1.0–1.6
HELICAL EXPOSURE TIME:	24–32 sec
RECONSTRUCTION INTERVAL:	2 mm (targeted to affected kidney)
SUPERIOR EXTENT:	1 cm superior to main renal arteries
INFERIOR EXTENT:	2 cm below UPJ

IV CONTRAST:

Concentration:	LOCM 300–350 mg I/mL or HOCM 282 mg I/mL
Rate:	5 mL/sec
Scan Delay:	30 sec for phase 1, 15 min for phase 2
Total Volume:	150 mL

COMMENTS:

1. Clamp nephrostomy tube (if present) when patient arrives to distend the renal pelvis for scanning.
2. Consider administering sterile saline via nephrostomy tube to distend the pelvocalyceal system in order to better differentiate the ureter from the renal pelvis.
3. Perform interactive interpretation on workstation using transaxial and MPR images.

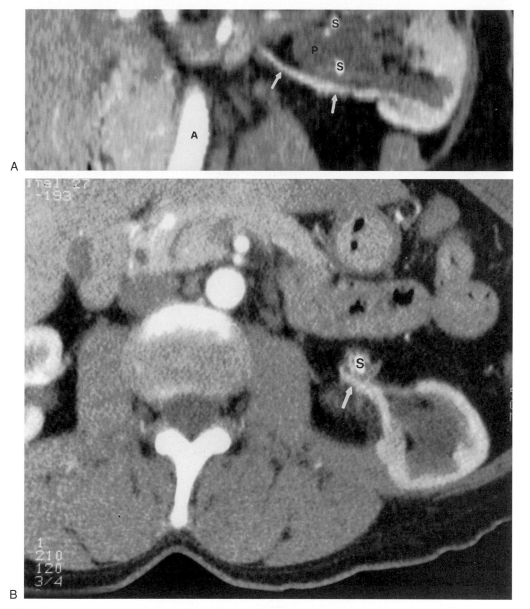

FIG. 14. Ureteropelvic junction obstruction with posterior crossing renal artery. Paracoronal (**A**) and transaxial (**B**) helical CT multiplanar reformations display 4-mm accessory lower pole left renal artery (*arrows*) crossing just posterior to the UPJ. Paracoronal reformation (**A**) clearly shows the vessel crossing the UPJ. However, the posterior position of this vessel relative to the UPJ is better shown on an orthogonal (transaxial) reformation in **B**. Ureteral stent is present within renal pelvis and proximal left ureter. P = renal pelvis; S = ureteral stent; A = aorta. (Reprinted with permission from Brink JA, McFarland EG, Heiken JP. Helical/spiral computed body tomography. *Clin Radiol* 1997;52:489–503.)

Protocol 15:
RENAL COLIC (Fig. 15)

INDICATION:	*Evaluation of patients with known or suspected renal or ureteral calculi as a cause for acute flank pain.*
SCANNER SETTINGS:	kVp: 120–140 mAs: 210–330
ORAL CONTRAST:	None
PHASE OF RESPIRATION:	Suspended expiration
SLICE THICKNESS:	5 mm
PITCH:	1.6
HELICAL EXPOSURE TIME:	24–32 sec
RECONSTRUCTION INTERVAL:	5 mm (2 mm in regions of concern with FOV targeted to suspicious regions)
SUPERIOR EXTENT:	Upper pole of kidneys
INFERIOR EXTENT:	Symphysis pubis
IV CONTRAST:	None
COMMENTS:	When calcifications are detected at the ureterovesical junction (UVJ), consider rescanning pelvis in prone position to distinguish mobile stones in the bladder from stones impacted at the UVJ.

FIG. 15. Left distal ureteral calculus. (**A,B**) Transaxial helical CT images performed without intravenous contrast material demonstrates proximal hydroureter (**A**, *arrow*) secondary to a distal left ureteral stone (**B**). Although not necessary in this case, a multiplanar reformation as shown in **C** may be helpful to confirm the intraureteral nature of such a calcification (*arrow* = ureter). (Reprinted with permission from Brink JA, McFarland EG, Heiken JP. Helical/spiral computed body tomography. *Clin Radiol* 1997;52:489–503.)

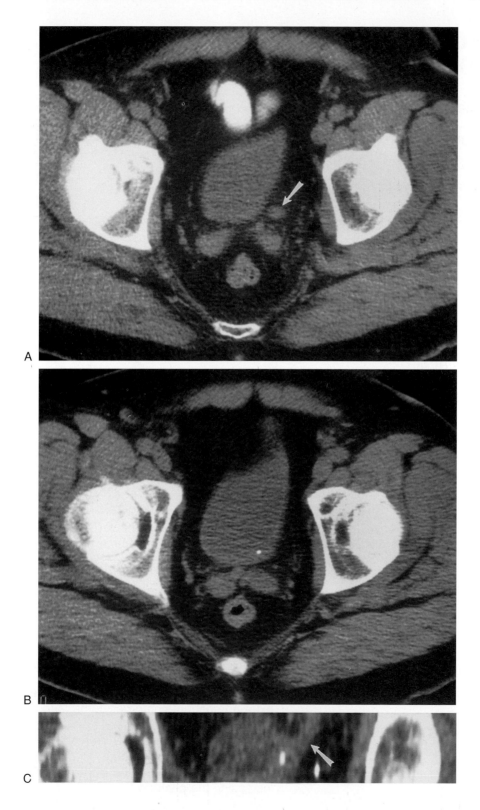

A

B

C

Protocol 16:
ADRENAL GLANDS (Fig. 16)

INDICATION:	*Rule out adrenal mass or hyperplasia*
SCANNER SETTINGS:	kVp: 120–140 mAs: 250–330
ORAL CONTRAST:	Optional, preferred
PHASE OF RESPIRATION:	Expiration after routine hyperventilation
SLICE THICKNESS:	3–5 mm
PITCH:	1.0–1.4
HELICAL EXPOSURE TIME:	15–30 sec
RECONSTRUCTION INTERVAL:	3–5 mm
SUPERIOR EXTENT:	Localizing scans are obtained to find the area just above the superior aspect of the adrenal glands
INFERIOR EXTENT:	Beneath the inferior border of the adrenal glands

IV CONTRAST:

Concentration:	LOCM 300–320 mg iodine/mL or HOCM 282 mg iodine/mL (60% solution)
Rate:	2–3 mL/sec
Scan Delay:	60–70 sec
Total Volume:	100–150 mL

COMMENTS:

1. To rule out pheochromocytoma, scans can usually be performed at 1-cm intervals. If adrenal glands are normal, scans to the aortic bifurcation organ of Zuckerkandl or even to the bladder should be performed to assess for extra-adrenal pheochromocytoma (see Protocol 17).
2. Thinner-section scans may be made in patients with MEA syndrome.
3. Length of coverage can be increased by increasing the pitch up to 2.0.

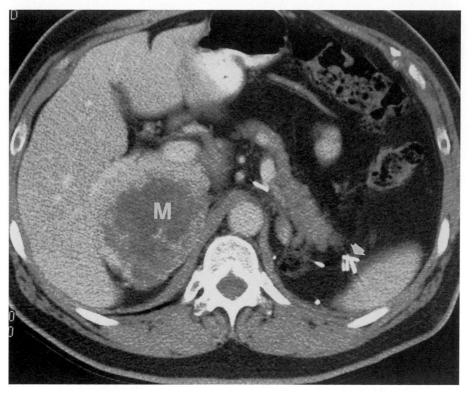

FIG. 16. Large inhomogenous mass in right adrenal (M). Necrotic metastasis in patient with malignant melanoma and previous resection of left adrenal mass, clips noted (*arrowhead*).

Protocol 17:
ADRENAL GLANDS (Fig. 17)

INDICATION:	*Suspected pheochromocytoma*
SCANNER SETTINGS:	kVp: 120 mAs: 250–330
ORAL CONTRAST:	600–800-mL oral contrast media given 45 min prior to the study. An additional 200 mL given just prior to scanning.
PHASE OF RESPIRATION:	Suspended inspiration
SLICE THICKNESS:	3–5 mm
PITCH:	1.0–1.4

HELICAL EXPOSURE TIME:	Single helical scan: 24–32 sec
	Multiple helical scans:
	  First scan duration: 10–20 sec
	  Breathing interval: 7–15 sec
	  2nd scan duration: 10–20 sec

RECONSTRUCTION INTERVAL:	3–5 mm
SUPERIOR EXTENT:	Just above upper poles of kidneys or top of adrenal glands, depending upon organs of interest.
INFERIOR EXTENT:	Aortic bifurcation (may continue to symphysis pubis if biochemical documentation is present but no mass is seen as a small percentage of pheochromocytomas may involve the bladder).

IV CONTRAST:

Concentration:	LOCM 300–320 mg iodine/mL or HOCM 282 mg iodine/mL (60% solution)
Note:	Uniphasic: 2–3 mL/sec
Scan Delay:	60 sec
Total Volume:	125 mL

COMMENTS:

1. IV contrast media may not be necessary for examinations of the adrenal glands.

2. The risk of a hypertensive crisis in a patient with a pheochromocytoma after IV administration of iodinated contrast media is not well documented in the literature, but it appears to be extremely low. If the radiologist is using IV contrast media in a patient with biochemical evidence of a pheochromocytoma, he or she should have phentolamine (an alpha-adrenergic blocker) available in case of a hypertensive reaction.

3. Length of coverage can be increased by increasing the pitch up to 2.0.

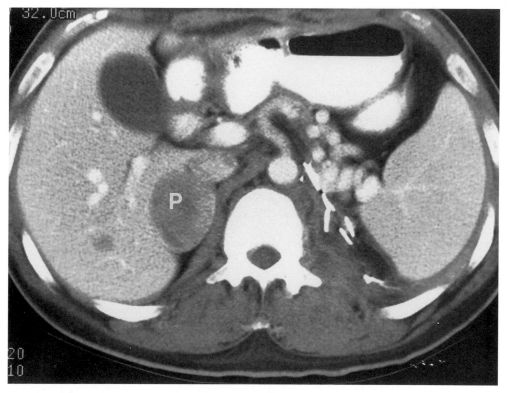

FIG. 17. Incidental pheochromocytoma (P) in patient with prior left nephrectomy for renal cell carcinoma and known metastatic disease.

Helical (Spiral) Computed Tomography,
edited by Paul M. Silverman.
Lippincott–Raven Publishers, Philadelphia © 1998.

5

Protocols for Helical CT of the Musculoskeletal System

Elliot K. Fishman

Department of Radiology, Johns Hopkins Hospital, Baltimore, Maryland 21287

The role of computed tomographic (CT) scanning in the evaluation of musculoskeletal pathology has had its peaks and valleys over the years. In the early to mid-1980s CT was the modality of choice for evaluating a wide range of musculoskeletal pathologies. However, with the introduction of clinical magnetic resonance imaging (MRI) the role of CT diminished and there appeared to be little interest in pursuing potential applications. With the advent of helical CT the interest in musculoskeletal applications has again increased (1–5). This is in great part related to the ability of helical CT to rapidly scan patients and to create volume data sets that can be used for highly detailed three-dimensional reconstructions. The impact of three-dimensional imaging is especially felt in orthopedic applications where clinical decision making is complex and treatment options vary.

The applications of CT in the musculoskeletal system can be divided into trauma, infection or inflammatory disease, those connected with oncology, and miscellaneous conditions (6–12). The most common application in our clinical practice is trauma. This makes up a substantial portion of our musculoskeletal CT work and not surprisingly is closely tied to multiplanar and three-dimensional imaging. We also do a significant number of cases of inflammatory disease because our population is heavily weighted toward immunosuppressed patients, whether due to bone marrow transplants or AIDS (3,13,14).

The advent of helical CT is making substantial differences in physicians' selection of radiologic examinations. In the musculoskeletal system the importance of a rapid diagnosis as well as a complete understanding and definition of extent of disease is something that helical CT can routinely provide. Helical CT can also provide this information in a very cost-effective manner in even the most uncooperative patients. The information obtained through CT is classically a critical part of patient management decisions.

APPLICATIONS

Trauma

Regardless of the anatomic area of involvement—be it the acetabulum and pelvis, spine, or wrist—CT plays a major role in patient diagnosis, triage, and management (15–26). The role of CT can typically be divided into cases where plain-film evaluation leaves the presence of a fracture somewhat in doubt and those where the diagnosis is made but CT is done to help plan surgery or select a more conservative management. This uncertainty could result from poor positioning of the patient, indeterminate radiographs, or disparity between the patient's symptoms and the radiographic findings. In these cases CT scanning can be done to determine whether a fracture is indeed present. In hospitals with a CT scanner in the emergency department this problem-solving role is easier to implement.

When performing musculoskeletal CT it is important to optimize the technical aspects of the examination. We routinely use helical CT with narrow collimation in the 2–3-mm range, depending on the body part studied. The reconstruction interval is typically 3 mm but can be 1 mm, particularly in areas such as the wrist, where thin-section and narrow-increment reconstruction is mandatory. These increased slices provide no additional radiation exposure to the patient but are critical in creating optimal data sets.

When evaluating musculoskeletal trauma we have found that reconstruction of images with the bone or high-resolution algorithm is most valuable. This algorithm will vary from scanner to scanner as well as between scanners of the same manufacturer. It is important to become familiar with your own system and choose the bone reconstruction algorithm that is best for you. The technical support staff of your equipment vendor may be helpful in letting you know which parameters are available and allowing you to select the one that is most appropriate.

Although in most cases intravenous contrast is not necessary when evaluating bony trauma, there are situations when it can become extremely important. For example, in pelvic injuries where vascular injury is suspected it is very helpful to do a helical CT using CT angiographic technique. In this process we can evaluate the aorta, iliac vessels and their branching, and the bony pelvis in a single examination. Similarly, in patients with sternal or sternoclavicular joint injury (27–34) it is important to not only evaluate the bony structures to define the extent of fracture and dislocation but also to obtain a vascular study to exclude injury to the aorta or great vessels. It is important to recognize that one of the advantages of this technique is that in many cases angiography can be avoided.

In choosing the scan parameters for a specific anatomic area several considerations play a role (35–38). The first is the area or volume that needs to be covered. If you are simply scanning the wrist, then narrow collimation in the range of 2 mm can be done with reconstructions at 1-mm intervals (39). The pitch can be in a range of 1–1.5. If, however, we need to scan a larger area, such as the femur or an area from the knee to the ankle, then we must make several compromises. In some cases we can use narrow collimation such as 3 mm but increase the pitch to 2 and cover a reasonable distance with the newer subsecond scanners. In other cases thicker-slice collimation of just 5 mm can be done to cover a longer distance. Initially, our experience was somewhat disappointing with using higher pitch in musculoskeletal imaging. Images were degraded by an element of noise and were less than satisfactory. With the newer scanners and their higher mAs settings as well as new bone reconstruction algorithms, this problem has apparently been resolved and helical CT is the study of choice.

An important aspect of musculoskeletal imaging, but particularly trauma imaging, is the use of reformatted images. These typically are categorized as multiplanar reconstruction and three-dimensional imaging. Multiplanar reconstruction (MPR) is the reformatting of data typically along the sagittal and coronal plane, although any off-axis can also be obtained. This is available on all scanners and typically takes several seconds to several minutes to perform. The advantage of helical CT with MPR is that it is cost effective and provides the clinician with images in any plane or perspective chosen. This is particularly valuable in supplementing the information provided by routine transaxial CT images. In our practice we routinely do these on all patients.

The second process revolves around three-dimensional imaging (40–45). A lot is being written about the various techniques used for three-dimensional imaging, including volume-rendering technique, shaded-surface technique, and maximum-intensity projection. Except for those cases with secondary vascular imaging, the key reconstruction algorithms used in musculoskeletal imaging are shaded-surface display and volume rendering.

We cannot discuss here the advantages of volume rendering and the limitations of shaded-surface techniques, but suffice it to say that three-dimensional imaging is progressing and will continue to become an even more important part of mainstream radiology. It has been our experience that three-dimensional reconstructions are especially valuable to the referring physician for them to understand the "personality of the injury." Orthopedic surgeons are advocates of this technique and find that it provides information that simple transaxial images do not. It is our feeling that the best way of looking at three-dimensional imaging is interactively in real time, and we have found this to be helpful in clinical practice.

Musculoskeletal Inflammation

With the ever-increasing numbers of immunosuppressed patients—whether those with a bone marrow transplant, high-dose steroid use for renal failure, or AIDS—we are seeing an increasing number of patients with the potential for musculoskeletal infection. Our experience has been that helical CT is a rapid and accurate technique for evaluating suspected or known musculoskeletal infection (46). The key parameters in these cases relate to the ability to scan the patient quickly while intravenous iodinated contrast is accentuating the difference between normal and abnormal structures such as those in muscle.

When intravenous (IV) contrast is not used but substantial inflammation is present, we can still usually detect the pathologic process. However, information regarding extent of inflammation and level of involvement is substantially inferior. Our protocols for contrast enhancement techniques are described in the specific protocols, but a few comments are in order. The use of intravenous contrast is to accentuate the difference between normal and abnormal tissue. When muscle becomes edematous or ischemic, it usually enlarges and has less sharp edges due to edema. However, particularly with older scanners, this may be easy to overlook, especially if comparison with the contralateral is not performed. With intravenous contrast we find that the normal musculature will enhance even up to 50–70 Hounsfield units (HU).

With helical CT we typically will scan at around 30–40 sec after we begin the injection of contrast. We have found this to be an ideal time to be able to optimize differentiation between normal and abnormal muscle. It should be noted that one of the potential limitations, at least from a theoretical perspective, is that enhancing muscle abscesses can look very similar to tumors. However, in most cases the clinical history is obviously different and the individual case is not typically problematic.

When evaluating muscle inflammation it is also important to obtain bone windows through the area of interest. Often bony involvement is a primary source of the inflammatory process or may become secondarily involved (14). This is particularly true in infection in the chest wall, especially around the sternoclavicular joint and the sternum.

In the evaluation of musculoskeletal infection we will typically image the patient with a standard algorithm. The high-resolution algorithm or bone algorithms create substantial noise, which makes the images suboptimal for viewing the soft tissues. In cases where high-resolution images of bone are desired, reconstruction with both algorithms is ideal.

In most cases of musculoskeletal inflammation three-dimensional or multiplanar imaging is not needed. However, in select cases it may be very valuable, particularly in determining the extent of inflammation that may be helpful to the surgeon in preoperative planning.

Musculoskeletal Tumors

Although MRI is the accepted study of choice for musculoskeletal tumors, the recent Radiology Diagnostic Oncology Group (RDOG) report showed little difference in staging between CT and MRI in the evaluation of musculoskeletal tumors. We have always found

CT to be valuable in looking at soft-tissuemasses, particularly by determining attenuation values (9,48–50). With CT it is very easy to determine if a lesion is a lipoma or if it is hemorrhagic. The extent of tumor can be well seen typically with CT, and as noted there is little difference statistically between it and MRI.

One of the most common oncologic uses for CT is in cases where there is suspected bony metastasis and there may be some discordance between clinical examination, radiographs, and bone scans. In these cases focused high-resolution CT scans can be done to determine if there is any bony involvement. In these cases thin collimation with narrow interscan spacing is very valuable. We also find that multiplanar reconstruction and three-dimensional imaging are very valuable, particularly when lesions involve areas near joint space and one is trying to determine whether the patient is in danger of pathologic fracture. Multiplanar reconstruction, particularly in the sagittal plane, is very valuable when looking at the acetabulum and lumbar spine and in determining the extent of pathology in these regions.

The role of CT in the evaluation of primary musculoskeletal tumors will vary from institution to institution. CT is excellent at defining the presence and type of matrix within a lesion as well as determining the extent of bony destruction. In terms of soft-tissue involvement with IV contrast and helical CT, we can get a good feel of the extent of tumor involvement. However, MRI does appear to be superior because of its direct multiplanar capabilities.

One interesting finding related to helical CT is the frequency of detection of musculoskeletal metastases as incidental findings. We have seen many cases of metastases to muscle presenting as hypervascular lesions ranging in size from 5 mm to 5 cm. In most cases the patients have not been symptomatic as a result of these lesions. The common tumors where we have found this to occur have been those resulting from lung cancer, renal cancer, and melanoma.

CONCLUSION

Helical CT provides unique opportunities for imaging the musculoskeletal system by providing the capabilities of high-quality volume data sets and the ability to optimally time contrast infusion and data acquisition. The continued development of three-dimensional imaging and multidimensional displays provides substantial advantages in musculoskeletal imaging. With the continued development of both CT technology and computer software the role of CT in musculoskeletal imaging will continue to expand in the near future.

REFERENCES

1. Dillon EH, van Leeuwen MS, Fernandez MA, Mali WPTM. Spiral CT angiography. *AJR* 1993;B160:1273–1278.
2. Fishman EK. Oncologic applications of spiral CT. In: Fishman EK, Jeffrey RB, eds. *Spiral CT: principles, techniques and clinical applications.* New York: Raven Press, 1995.
3. Fishman EK. Spiral CT evaluation of the musculoskeletal system. In: Fishman EK, Jeffrey RB, eds. *Spiral CT: principles, techniques and clinical applications.* New York: Raven Press, 1995.
4. Pretorius ES, Fishman EK. Helical (spiral) CT of the musculoskeletal system. *Radiol Clin North Am* 1995; 33(5):949–979.
5. Pretorius ES, Scott WW Jr, Fishman EK. Acute trauma of the shoulder: role of spiral CT imaging. *Emerg Radiol* 1995;2(1):13–17.
6. Brueton LA, Dillon MJ, Winter RM. Ellis-van Creveld syndrome, Jeune syndrome, and renal-hepatic pancreatic dysplasia: separate entities or disease spectrum? *J Med Genet* 1990;27:252–255.
7. Coumas JM, Waite RJ, Goss TP, Ferrari DA, Kanzaria PK, Pappas AM. CT and MR evaluation of the labral capsular ligamentous complex of the shoulder. *AJR* 1992;158:591–597.
8. Kozlowski K, Masel J. Asphyxiating thoracic dystrophy without respiratory disease. *Pediatr Radiol* 1976;5:30.
9. Ma LD, Frassica FJ, Scott WW Jr, Fishman EK, Zerhouni EA. Differentiation of benign and malignant musculoskeletal tumors: potential pitfalls with MR imaging. *Radiographics* 1995;15:349–366.
10. Oberklaid F, Danks DM, Mayne V, Campbell P. Asphyxiating thoracic dysplasia: clinical, radiological and pathological information on 10 patients. *Arch Dis Child* 1977;52:758–765.
11. Olson PN, Everson LI, Griffiths HJ. Staging of musculoskeletal tumors. *Radiol Clin North Am* 1994;32(1): 151–162.
12. Rabassa AE, Guinto FC Jr, Crow WN, Chaljub G, Wright GD, Storey GS. CT of the spine: value of reformatted images. *AJR* 1993;161:1223–1227.

13. Beauchamp NJ, Scott WW Jr, Gottlieb LM, Fishman EK. CT evaluation of soft tissue muscle infection and inflammation: a systematic compartmental approach. *Skeletal Radiol* 1995;24:317–324.
14. Schauwecker DS, Braunstein EM, Wheat LJ. Diagnostic imaging of osteomyelitis. *Infect Dis Clin North Am* 1990;4(3):441–463.
15. Dias JJ, Stirling A, Finlay D, et al. Computerized axial tomography for tibial plateau fractures. *J Bone Joint Surg* 1987;69B:84–88.
16. Friedman L, Johnson GH, Yong-Hing K. Computed tomography of wrist trauma. *J Can Assoc Radiol* 1990; 41:141–145.
17. Munk PL, Connell DG, Vellet AD. Computed tomography of the knee. *Can Assoc Radiol J* 1991;42(6):397–405.
18. Newberg AH. Computed tomography of joint injuries. *Radiol Clin North Am* 1990;28(2):445–460.
19. Passariello R, Trecco F, dePaulis F, Masciocchi C, Bonnani G, Zobel B. Meniscal lesions of the knee joint: CT diagnosis. *Radiology* 1985;157:29–34.
20. Pitt MJ, Lund PJ, Speer DP. Imaging of the pelvis and hip. *Orthop Clin North Am* 1990;21(3):545–559.
21. Pitt MJ, Ruth JT, Benjamin JB. Trauma to the pelvic ring and acetabulum. *Semin Roentgenol* 1992;27(4): 299–318.
22. Schlesinger AE, Hernandez RJ. Disease of the musculoskeletal system in children: imaging with CT, sonography, and MR. *AJR* 1992;158:729–741.
23. Tile M (moderator), Helfet DL, Kellam JF, Letournel E, Matta JM. Symposium: management of acetabular fractures part I. *Contemp Orthop* 1992;25(3):301–324.
24. Wadlington VR, Hendrix RW, Rogers LF. Computed tomography of posterior fracture-dislocations of the shoulder: case reports. *J Trauma* 1992;32(1):113–115.
25. Wilson AJ, Totty WG, et al. Shoulder joint: arthrographic CT and long-term follow-up, with surgical correlation. *Radiology* 1989;173:329–333.
26. Blum A, Boyer B, Regent D, Simon JM, Claudon M, Mole D. Direct coronal view of the shoulder with arthrographic CT. *Radiology* 1993;188:677–681.
27. Burnstein MI, Pozniak MA. Computed tomography with stress maneuver to demonstrate sternoclavicular joint dislocation. *J Comput Assist Tomogr* 1990;14(1):159–160.
28. Cope R, Riddervold HO. Posterior dislocation of the sternoclavicular joint: report of two cases, with emphasis on radiologic management and early diagnosis. *Skeletal Radiol* 1988;17:247–250.
29. Keogh P, Masterson E, Murphy B, McCoy CT, Gibney RG, Kelly E. The role of radiography and computed tomography in the diagnosis of acute dislocation of the proximal tibiofibular joint. *Br J Radiol* 1993;66(782): 108–111.
30. Davies AM. Review: the current role of computed tomographic arthrography of the shoulder. *Clin Radiol* 1991; 44:369–375.
31. Habibian A, Stauffer A, Resnick D, Reicher MA, et al. Comparison of conventional and computed arthrotomography with MR imaging in the evaluation of the shoulder. *J Comput Assist Tomogr* 1989;13(6):968–975.
32. Hunter JC, Blatz DJ, Escobedo EM. SLAP lesions of the glenoid labrum: CT arthrographic and arthroscopic correlation. *Radiology* 1992;184:513–518.
33. Kilcoyne RF, Shuman WP, et al. The Neer classification of displaced proximal humeral fractures: spectrum of findings on plain radiographs and CT scans. *AJR* 1990;154(5):1029–1033.
34. Scott WW Jr, Fishman EK, Magid D. Acetabular fractures: optimal imaging. *Radiology* 1987;165:537–539.
35. Kalender WA. Technical foundations of spiral CT. *Semin Ultrasound CT MR* 1994;15(2):81–89.
36. Kuszyk BS, Fishman EK. Direct coronal CT of the wrist: helical acquisition with simplified patient positioning. *AJR* 1996;166:419–420.
37. Ney DR, Fishman EK, Kawashima A, et al. Comparison of helical and serial CT with regard to three-dimensional imaging of musculoskeletal anatomy. *Radiology* 1992;185:865–869.
38. Reiser M, Rupp N, Karpf M, Feuerbach ST, Anacker H. Evaluation of the cruciate ligaments by CT. *Eur J Radiol* 1981;1:9–15.
39. Stewart NR, Gilula LA. CT of the wrist: a tailored approach. *Radiology* 1992;183:13–20.
40. Billet FP, Schmitt WG, Gay B. Computed tomography in traumatology with special regard to the advances of three dimensional display. *Arch Orthop Trauma Surg* 1992;111(3):131–137.
41. Fishman EK, Magid D, Ney D, et al. Three-dimensional imaging. *Radiology* 1991;181:321–327.
42. Kuhlman JE, Fishman EK, Scott WW Jr, Magid D, Siegelman SS. Two-dimensional and three-dimensional evaluation of the painful shoulder. *Orthop Rev* 1989;18:1201–1208.
43. Kuszyk BS, Ney DR, Fishman EK. The current state of the art in three-dimensional oncologic imaging: an overview. *Int J Radiat Oncol Biol Phys* 1995;33(5):1029–1039.
44. Kuszyk BS, Heath DG, Bliss DF, Fishman EK. Skeletal 3D CT: advantages of volume rendering over surface rendering. *Skeletal Radiol* 1996;25:207–214.
45. Ney DR, Fishman EK, Magid D, Robertson DD, Kawashima A. Three-dimensional volumetric display of CT data: effect of scan parameters upon image quality. *J Comput Assist Tomogr* 1991;15(5):875–885.
46. Magid D, Fishman EK. Musculoskeletal infections in patients with AIDS: CT findings. *AJR* 1992;158:603–607.
47. Tecce PM, Fishman EK. Spiral CT with multiplanar reconstruction in the diagnosis of sternoclavicular osteomyelitis. *Skeletal Radiol* 1995;24:275–281.
48. Magid D. Two-dimensional and three-dimensional computed tomographic imaging in musculoskeletal tumors. *Radiol Clin North Am* 1993;31(2):425–447.
49. Manaster, BJ. Musculoskeletal oncologic imaging. *Int J Radiat Biol Phys* 1991;21:1643–1651.
50. Murphy WA Jr. Imaging bone tumors in the 1990s. *Cancer* 1991;67(4 suppl):1169–1176.

Protocol 1:
ACETABULUM AND HIP JOINT (Fig. 1)

INDICATION:	*Trauma/fractures*
SCANNER SETTINGS:	kVp: 120 mAs: 280
ORAL CONTRAST:	None
PHASE OF RESPIRATION:	Inspiration
SLICE THICKNESS:	3 mm
PITCH:	1.0–2.0
HELICAL EXPOSURE TIME:	30 sec
RECONSTRUCTION INTERVAL:	3 mm
SUPERIOR EXTENT:	Mid-body pelvis
INFERIOR EXTENT:	Inferior aspect of symphysis pubis
IV CONTRAST:	None
COMMENTS:	1. This protocol is used both for detection of fracture as well as defining extent. 2. Reconstruction at bone algorithm is helpful. 3. Multiplanar (especially sagittal) and three-dimensional imaging is critical in these patients. 4. IV contrast can be used for CT angiography. 5. Pelvic vascular injury is suspected.

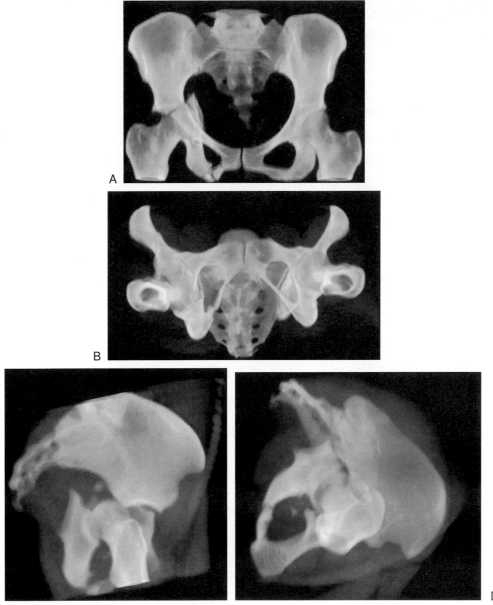

FIG. 1. (**A,B**) Complex right acetabular fracture and dislocation. Select views define the extent of the fracture with dislocation posteriorly. Note the ability to use three-dimensional reconstructions with edited views (**C,D**) to define the full extent of injury as well as location of joint fragments. These views are particularly helpful for preoperative planning.

Protocol 2:
PELVIS (Fig. 2)

INDICATION:	*Trauma*
SCANNER SETTINGS:	kVp: 120 mAs: 280
ORAL CONTRAST:	None
PHASE OF RESPIRATION:	Inspiration
SLICE THICKNESS:	3 mm
PITCH:	1.0–1.5
HELICAL EXPOSURE TIME:	30–40 sec
RECONSTRUCTION INTERVAL:	3 mm
SUPERIOR EXTENT:	Top of iliac crest
INFERIOR EXTENT:	Symphysis pubis
IV CONTRAST:	Usually none needed
COMMENTS:	1. This protocol is used when complex pelvic pathology is present and injury to the SI joints, sacrum, or iliac wing are suspected in addition to acetabular injuries. 2. Three-dimensional and MPR imaging is critical. 3. IV contrast may be used if concurrent vascular injury is suspected.

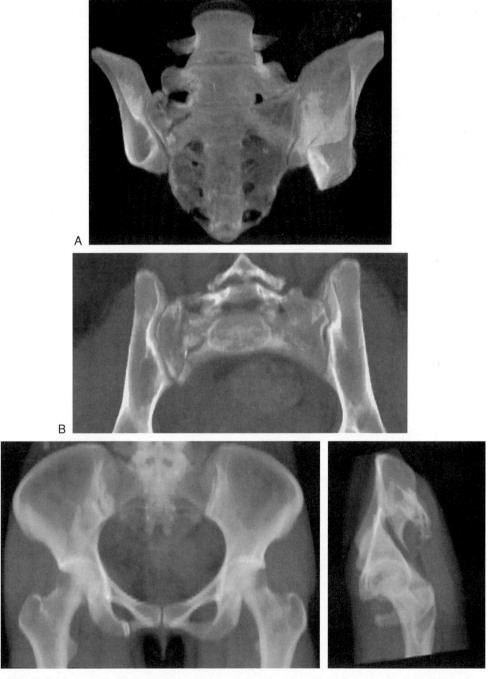

FIG. 2. (**A,B**) Sacral fracture. Select views in three-dimensional format clearly define the fracture through the right sacral elements. This fracture was not seen on plain x-rays. (**C,D**) Iliac wing fracture. Select three-dimensional views with editing are optimal for defining the fracture that was harder to detect on the three-dimensional view (and plain x-ray) in AP projection.

Protocol 3:
WRIST (Fig. 3)

INDICATION:	*Trauma*
SCANNER SETTINGS:	kVp: 120 mAs: 280
ORAL CONTRAST:	None
PHASE OF RESPIRATION:	Patient must remain motionless
SLICE THICKNESS:	2 mm
PITCH:	1.0–1.5
HELICAL EXPOSURE TIME:	20–25 sec
RECONSTRUCTION INTERVAL:	1 mm
SUPERIOR EXTENT:	Superior aspect of hand
INFERIOR EXTENT:	Inferior aspect of hand
IV CONTRAST:	None

COMMENTS:

1. Place the patient behind the scanner and have them place their hand in the scanning gantry with the hand placed parallel to the x-ray beam. Several test runs are done to make sure the patient is not surprised by the table motion and neither helps nor hinders table movement.
2. The high-resolution algorithm is needed in these cases.

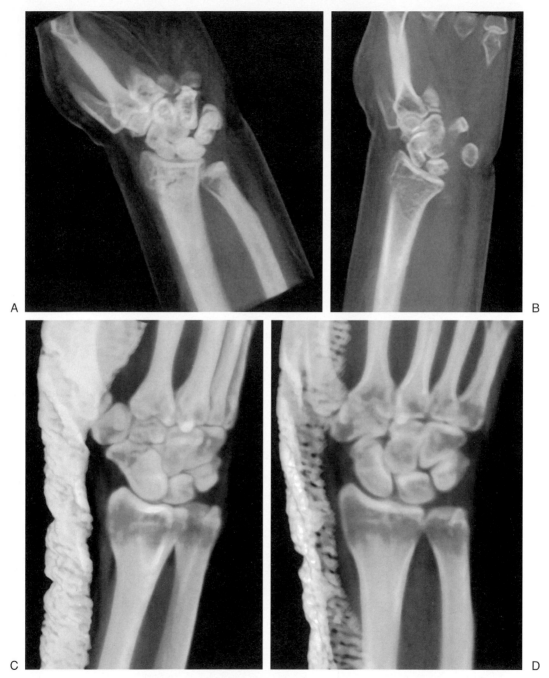

FIG. 3. (**A,B**) Impacted fracture of the distal radius. Use of three-dimensional reconstruction with interactive editing allows one to carefully define the full extent of injury. (**C,D**) Scaphoid fracture. The ability to use various transparencies for 3-D is helpful in defining the extent of scaphoid fractures. The study can be performed either to determine the presence of fracture or define healing.

Protocol 4:
KNEE (Fig. 4)

INDICATION:	*Trauma*
SCANNER SETTINGS:	kVp: 120 mAs: 280
ORAL CONTRAST:	None
PHASE OF RESPIRATION:	Patient must remain still during the study
SLICE THICKNESS:	2–3 mm
PITCH:	1.0–2.0
HELICAL EXPOSURE TIME:	Up to 30 sec
RECONSTRUCTION INTERVAL:	1–2 mm
SUPERIOR EXTENT:	2 cm above suspected fracture
INFERIOR EXTENT:	2 cm below suspected fracture
IV CONTRAST:	None
COMMENTS:	Coronal and sagittal reconstructions are valuable in these cases.

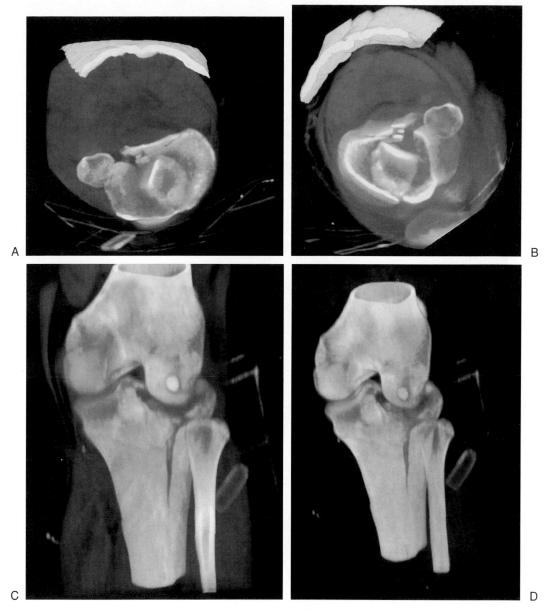

FIG. 4. (**A,B**) Tibial plateau fracture. Three-dimensional reconstructions in multiple planes demonstrate the value of combining helical CT and imaging computing. The impaction of the femoral condyle on the tibial plateau is well understood from these views (**C,D**).

Protocol 5:
SHOULDER (Fig. 5)

INDICATION:	*Trauma*
SCANNER SETTINGS:	kVp: 120 mAs: 280
ORAL CONTRAST:	None
PHASE OF RESPIRATION:	Suspended respiration
SLICE THICKNESS:	3 mm
PITCH:	1.0–1.5
HELICAL EXPOSURE TIME:	30–40 sec
RECONSTRUCTION INTERVAL:	3 mm
SUPERIOR EXTENT:	Just above acromioclavicular joint
INFERIOR EXTENT:	Depending on the case the lower aspect may be as far as the scapular tip
IV CONTRAST:	Not routinely
COMMENTS:	1. Perform study with patients arms by their side. 2. Target reconstruction to the injured shoulder.

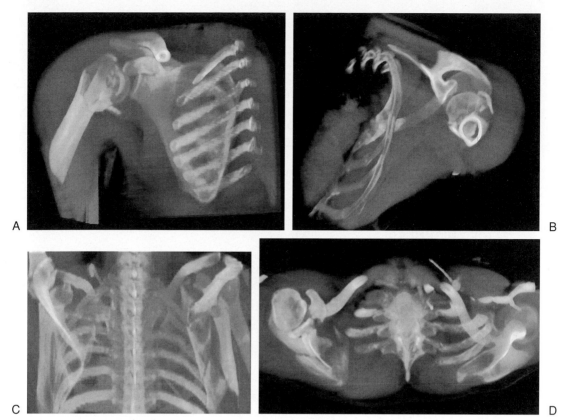

FIG. 5. (**A,B**) Complex fracture of the humeral head. Three-dimensional reconstructions demonstrate through varying obliquities the full extent of injury with impaction and fragmentation. (**C,D**) Three-dimensional reconstructions of a complex fracture of the left scapula. Scapula fractures are often missed on plain radiographs but can be well defined with CT imaging. Helical CT is very useful in the traumatized patient.

Protocol 6:
SPINE (Fig. 6)

INDICATION:	*Trauma*
SCANNER SETTINGS:	kVp: 120 mAs: 280
ORAL CONTRAST:	None
PHASE OF RESPIRATION:	Suspended inspiration
SLICE THICKNESS:	3 mm
PITCH:	1.0–2.0 (depending on size of area to be scanned)
HELICAL EXPOSURE TIME:	30–40 sec
RECONSTRUCTION INTERVAL:	2–3 mm
SUPERIOR EXTENT:	2–3 cm above area in question
INFERIOR EXTENT:	2–3 cm below area in question
IV CONTRAST:	Usually none
COMMENTS:	1. Multiplanar imaging, especially sagittal views, are very helpful in defining the extent of spinal trauma. 2. The scans are reconstructed with a high-resolution bone algorithm.

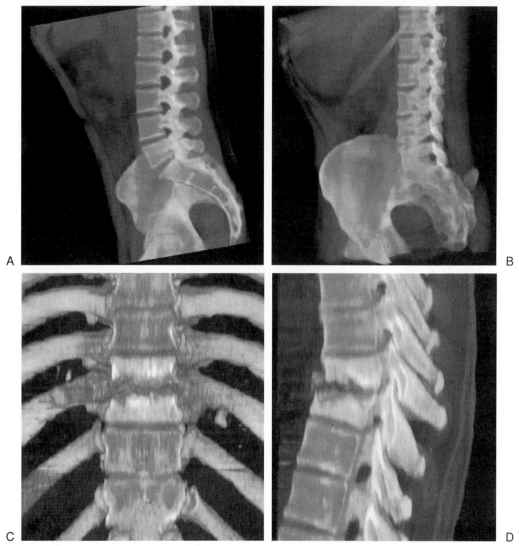

FIG. 6. (A,B) Normal lumbar spine. Three-dimensional reconstructions of suspected spinal fracture demonstrate no evidence of fracture. The details of the foramen, including the Scotty dog, are well seen on these views. **(C,D)** Osteomyelitis of the spine. In addition to evaluating trauma, CT with three-dimensional is excellent for looking at infection. Note the joint space and bone destruction on these images.

Protocol 7:
THREE-DIMENSIONAL ORTHOPEDIC
RECONSTRUCTION (Fig. 7)

INDICATION: *Usually for trauma*

SCANNER SETTINGS: kVp: 120
                             mAs: 280

ORAL CONTRAST: N/A

PHASE OF RESPIRATION: Patient must remain motionless

SLICE THICKNESS: 3 mm

PITCH: 1.0–1.3

HELICAL EXPOSURE TIME: 30–40 sec

**RECONSTRUCTION   1–2 mm
  INTERVAL:**

SUPERIOR EXTENT: 2 cm above area in question

INFERIOR EXTENT: 2 cm below area in question

IV CONTRAST: Usually not needed

COMMENTS: 1. Three-dimensional imaging can be done with
                              shaded-surface technique (SSD) or volume
                              rendering technique (VRT). We prefer the
                              accuracy of VRT.
                            2. Interactive three-dimensional is ideal with the
                              freedom to select any arbitrary view.

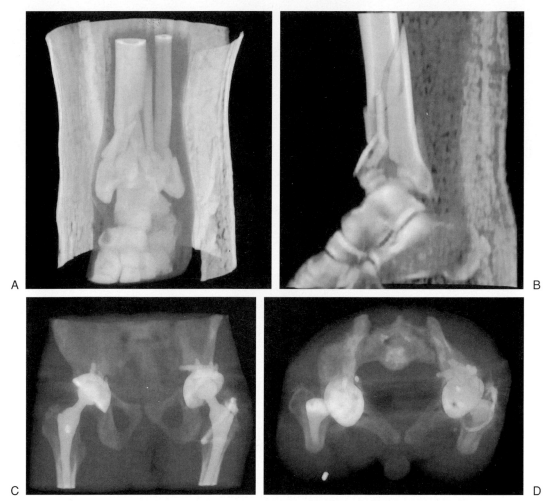

FIG. 7. (A,B) Distal tibia and fibula fracture. Three-dimensional reconstructions define the extent of the fracture and its fragmentation. **(C,D)** Loosening and rotation of left hip prosthesis. Despite significant artifact on routine transaxial CT images, three-dimensional reconstructions are valuable in evaluating patients with total hip prosthesis. In this case notice the rotation and poor position of the left acetabular cup. Note the lack of artifact.

Protocol 8:
STERNOCLAVICULAR JOINT (Fig. 8)

INDICATION: *Suspected infection*

SCANNER SETTINGS: kVp: 120
                          mAs: 280

ORAL CONTRAST: None

PHASE OF RESPIRATION: Suspended inspiration

SLICE THICKNESS: 3 mm

PITCH: 1.0

HELICAL EXPOSURE TIME: 25–30 sec

**RECONSTRUCTION
   INTERVAL:**   2–3 mm

SUPERIOR EXTENT: 2 cm above sternoclavicular joint

INFERIOR EXTENT: Mid-sternum

IV CONTRAST: See comments

COMMENTS: If the study is done to look for bony erosion only,
                          then a noncontrast high-resolution study is
                          satisfactory. However, since a soft-tissue
                          component as well as a mediastinal component
                          may be involved, we recommend using IV
                          contrast. We inject 2 mL/sec for a total of
                          100–120 mL.

FIG. 8. (**A,B**) Suspected infection of the sternoclavicular joint. Helical CT with three-dimensional reconstructions was done to evaluate suspected infection in this patient following coronary artery bypass surgery. This study does demonstrate the diasthesis of the medial stenotomy with some breakage of the lower bands. Even in sicker patients the speed of helical CT scanning allows studies to be successfully performed. (**C,D**) Sternoclavicular joint infection with muscle involvement. Two examples of intramuscular abscesses associated with sternoclavicular joint infection.

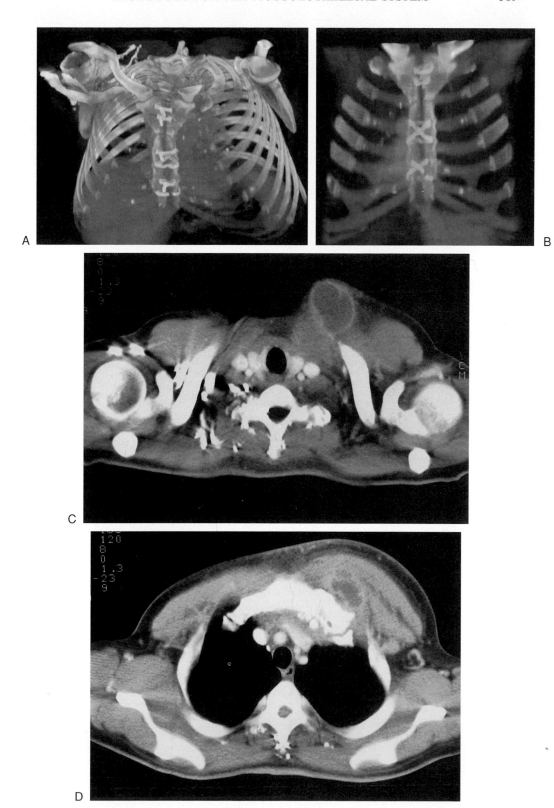

Protocol 9:
SUSPECTED OSTEOID OSTEOMA (Fig. 9)

INDICATION: *Tumor*

SCANNER SETTINGS: kVp: 120
                             mAs: 280

ORAL CONTRAST: None

PHASE OF RESPIRATION: Depending on location of the suspected lesion
                             the patient either remains still (i.e., femur) or
                             holds their breath (i.e., rib)

SLICE THICKNESS: 2 mm

PITCH: 1.5–2.0

HELICAL EXPOSURE TIME: Varies but usually 25–30 sec

RECONSTRUCTION   1–2 mm
INTERVAL:

SUPERIOR EXTENT: Above sclerotic zone on topogram/scout view

INFERIOR EXTENT: Beneath sclerotic zone on topogram/scout view

IV CONTRAST: None

COMMENTS: 1. Very wide window settings are needed to
                                detect the nidus. The dense sclerotic bone
                                may make this hard to find without the correct
                                window width/level settings.
                             2. CT can be used for guidance for RF
                                destruction of the lesion.

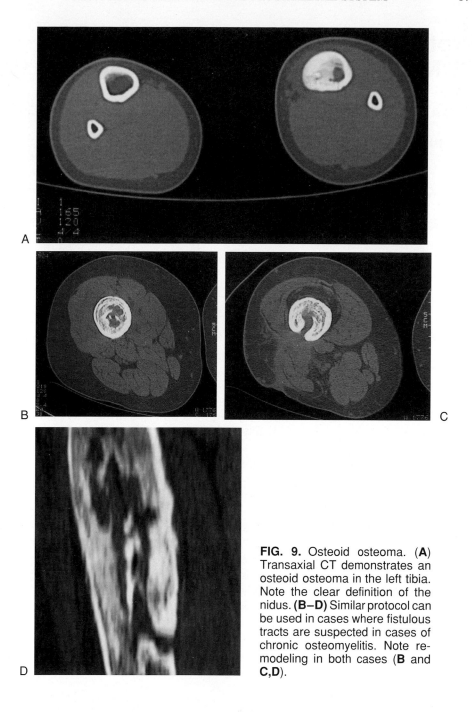

FIG. 9. Osteoid osteoma. (**A**) Transaxial CT demonstrates an osteoid osteoma in the left tibia. Note the clear definition of the nidus. (**B–D**) Similar protocol can be used in cases where fistulous tracts are suspected in cases of chronic osteomyelitis. Note remodeling in both cases (**B** and **C,D**).

Protocol 10:
CONGENITAL HIP DISLOCATION (Fig. 10)

INDICATION: *Congenital abnormality/post reduction study*

SCANNER SETTINGS: kVp: 120
                             mAs: 140–210

ORAL CONTRAST: None

PHASE OF RESPIRATION: Have the patient remain motionless. Sedation is
                             not needed.

SLICE THICKNESS: 3–4 mm

PITCH: 1.5

HELICAL EXPOSURE TIME: Usually 15 sec

RECONSTRUCTION   3 mm
  INTERVAL:

SUPERIOR EXTENT: Depending on the extent of surgery, it may begin
                             anywhere from the iliac crest downward.

INFERIOR EXTENT: Beneath the ischium

IV CONTRAST: None

COMMENTS: The study is done to limit the x-ray dose to the
                             child. Some institutions will only do a few select
                             images but this is better as we can generate
                             three-dimensional views. The inlet view on three-
                             dimensional is especially valuable in our
                             experience.

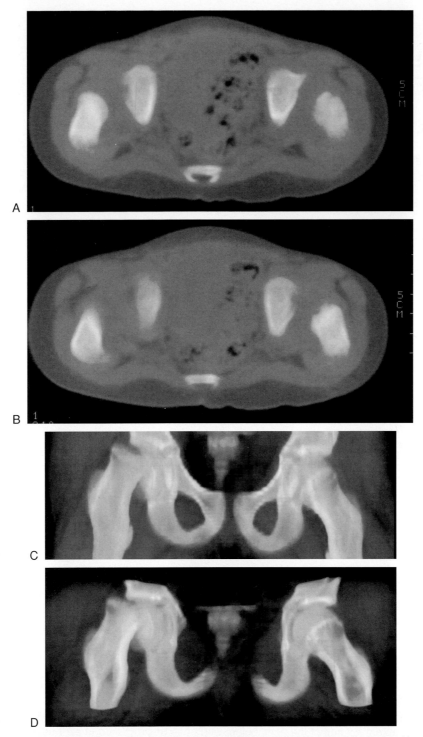

FIG. 10. (A,B) Congenital hip dislocation. Transaxial views demonstrate the malposition of the femoral heads relative to the acetabular joint space in this patient with congenital hip dislocations. A limited study through the hips can be done in these cases with helical CT. **(C,D)** Slipped capital femoral epiphyses (SCFE). CT is also valuable in defining the presence and extent of SCFE. It can also be used to determine the success of reduction.

Protocol 11:
SOFT-TISSUE MASS (Fig. 11)

INDICATION:	*Tumor, inflammatory*
SCANNER SETTINGS:	kVp: 120 mAs: 280
ORAL CONTRAST:	None
PHASE OF RESPIRATION:	Suspended respiration
SLICE THICKNESS:	5 mm
PITCH:	1.0
HELICAL EXPOSURE TIME:	30–40 sec
RECONSTRUCTION INTERVAL:	3–5 mm
SUPERIOR EXTENT:	2–4 cm above suspected lesion
INFERIOR EXTENT:	2–4 cm below suspected lesion

IV CONTRAST:

Concentration:	LOCM 350 mg I/mL or Hocm 282 MgI/ml (60% solution)
Total Volume:	120 mL
Injection rate:	2.5 mL/sec

COMMENTS: A 40-sec delay is usually satisfactory.

FIG. 11. (**A,B**) Aneurysmal bone cyst of the symphysis pubis. Large lytic lesion involves the pubis and anterior column of the acetabulum with bone destruction and expansion and a soft-tissue mass. (**C,D**) Femoral artery pseudoaneurysm following graft. Precontrast and helical study demonstrates that the mass palpated in the patient's thigh was a pseudoaneurysm following graft repair.

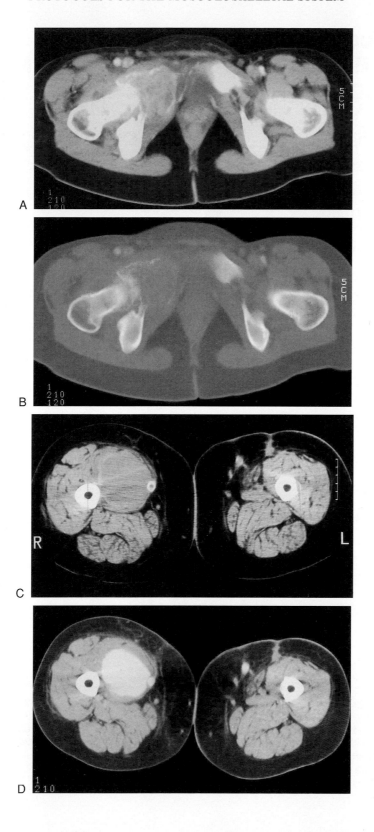

Protocol 12:
SUSPECTED METASTASES TO BONE
(Fig. 12)

INDICATION:	*Tumor, metastases*
SCANNER SETTINGS:	kVp: 120 mAs: 280
ORAL CONTRAST:	None
PHASE OF RESPIRATION:	Suspended respiration
SLICE THICKNESS:	3 mm
PITCH:	1.0
HELICAL EXPOSURE TIME:	20–40 sec
RECONSTRUCTION INTERVAL:	2–3 mm
SUPERIOR EXTENT:	2 cm above suspected lesion
INFERIOR EXTENT:	2 cm below suspected lesion
IV CONTRAST:	None
COMMENTS:	High-resolution algorithms are best for these cases.

FIG. 12. (A,B) Metastatic breast cancer to bone. Three-dimensional reconstructions demonstrate a lytic lesion in the superior portion of the right acetabulum. The patient had a history of breast cancer. The study defines the presence of the lesion as well as its extent, which can be used for either surgical planning or radiation therapy planning. **(C,D)** Myositis ossificans. Three-dimensional reconstructions for evaluation of a suspected muscular mass demonstrate an osteoid-like tumor arising off bone. Note the clear linear line extending between the mass and bone. This was not a primary tumor but was due to myositis ossificans.

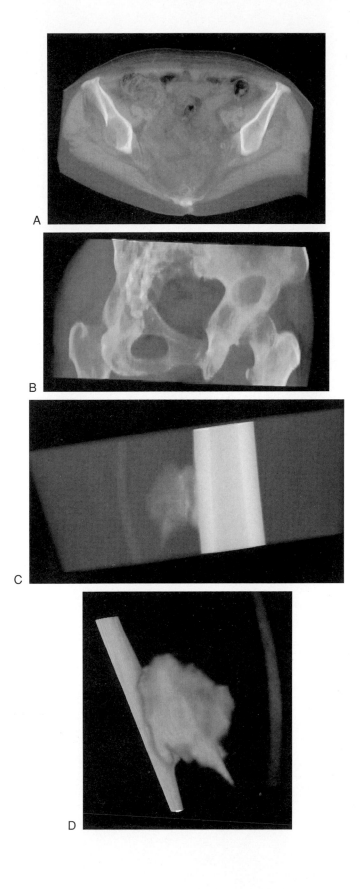

Helical (Spiral) Computed Tomography,
edited by Paul M. Silverman.
Lippincott–Raven Publishers, Philadelphia © 1998.

6

Protocols for Helical CT in Pediatrics

Marilyn J. Siegel

*Department of Radiology, Mallinckrodt Institute of Radiology, Washington University
School of Medicine, St. Louis, Missouri 63110*

Helical CT has a number of advantages in pediatric patients (1,2). First, the reconstruction capabilities it affords can improve lesion detection without increasing radiation exposure. Second, the helical examination, which is completed more rapidly than conventional CT studies, can eliminate or at least minimize motion artifacts. Third, the rapid imaging time can decrease the length of sedation and in some patients even the need for sedation. Finally, the relatively short scanning time allows contrast-enhanced scans to be performed during peak vascular enhancement. This is important in children because small volumes of intravenous contrast medium are being administered. This chapter presents some current applications of helical CT in pediatric patients and guidelines for performing these examinations.

TECHNIQUE

Sedation

Even though imaging time is shortened with helical CT, image degradation by patient motion remains a problem in young children. Children under 5 years of age usually require parenteral sedation. The drugs most commonly used in this age group are oral chloral hydrate and intravenous pentobarbital sodium (3,4). Children under 18 months of age usually receive oral chloral hydrate, 50–100 mg/kg, to a maximum dosage of 2000 mg. Patients 18 months of age and older are given intravenous pentobarbital sodium, 5 mg/kg, up to a maximum dose of 200 mg. A dose of 2.5 mg/kg is given initially as a slow bolus over 1–2 min. In most children, this dose of pentobarbital sodium is adequate. If sedation is unsuccessful, an additional dose of 1.25 mg/kg may be given after a 1–2-min delay. This same dose may be repeated 1–2 min later if necessary. The major advantages of intravenous barbiturate are its rapid action and a relatively short recovery time.

Other methods of sedation include rectal barbiturate and a combination of meperidine, chlorpromazine, and promethazine (known as a cardiac cocktail). The higher failure rates and prolonged duration of action are limitations of these drugs. In addition, the risks of respiratory and cardiac depression from the narcotic analgesics (e.g., meperidine) are significantly greater than the risks from oral chloral hydrate and the barbiturates. Therefore most examiners prefer the latter drugs. Regardless of the choice of drug, the use of parenteral sedation necessitates continuous monitoring and maintaining adequate cardiorespiratory support during and after the procedure.

When sedation is needed, the child should receive no solid foods for 6 hr and no liquids for 3 hr prior to the study. Children who are not to be sedated should be given nothing by mouth for 3 hr prior to the examination. This precaution is taken to reduce the risk of aspiration if nausea and vomiting occur during administration of intravenous contrast material.

After being sedated, the patient is placed on the CT table. The arms routinely are positioned above the head to eliminate streak artifacts and to provide an easily accessible route for administration of intravenous contrast.

Children older than 5 years of age usually will cooperate for CT studies after verbal reassurance and explanation of the procedure. The presence of a parent in the CT suite during the study is helpful to reassure and comfort the child.

Intravenous Contrast Medium

Nearly all CT examinations of the chest, abdomen, and pelvis are performed with intravenous contrast material. If contrast material is to be given, an intravenous catheter should be in place when the child arrives in the CT suite. This avoids the agitation and consequent patient motion that would otherwise be associated with venipuncture performed immediately prior to administering contrast material. The gauge of butterfly needle or intravenous cannula will vary with patient size, but the largest possible one should be placed.

If intravenous access is through a butterfly needle or central venous catheter, hand injection of contrast medium is recommended. A power injector is used in children who have antecubital cannulas (22 gauge or larger) in place (5). The rate of contrast injection is determined by the size of the catheter (Table 1). During the initial seconds of injection, the injection site should be carefully monitored for contrast extravasation. With appropriate selection of injection rates and patient monitoring, the use of a power injector is safe in children. Either low-osmolar-contrast (280–320 mg I/mL) or high-osmolar-contrast (282 mg I/mL) media can be used for CT examinations. The usual dose of contrast is 2 mL/kg up to a maximum of 4 mL/kg or 150 mL.

Optimal enhancement is a result of the rate of contrast administration, the total volume of contrast, and the timing between the injection of contrast and the onset of scanning. Most imaging strategies for helical CT have addressed optimization of hepatic enhancement (6–9). In children under 45 kg body weight, CT scanning of the abdomen using a power injector for contrast administration should begin after 100% of the contrast medium has been injected (8). It is more difficult to make recommendations for scan initiation using hand injections, because of variations in flow rates. Empirically, scanning should begin after 80% to 100% of the contrast material has been injected. The injection time with larger-gauge catheters (18–20 gauge) is faster than that for smaller-gauge catheters, and onset of scanning can be delayed until 100% of the contrast has been given. With smaller butterfly needles (22–24 gauge), scanning should begin sooner (after 80% to 90% of injected volume). The goal of both power and hand injection protocols is to scan higher on the liver enhancement curve and to avoid scanning at or after equilibrium. There are two exceptions to the preceding approach for contrast administration. First, scanning in neonates and very small children

TABLE 1. *Rate of contrast injection versus needle size*

Needle size (g)	Flow rate
22	1.2 mL/sec
20	1.5 mL/sec
18	2.0 mL/sec

should be delayed at least 30 sec to ensure that there is enhancement of the portal venous system. Second, children who weigh more than 45 kg can be scanned using adult protocols.

With hypervascular hepatic lesions, such as hemangioendotheliomas, there can be an advantage to imaging the liver twice, once during the arterial phase and once during the portal venous enhancement phase (10). This technique, also known as dual-phase imaging, requires a flow rate of at least 2 mL/sec and a monophasic injection. The arterial scan usually begins 10–15 sec after initiation of the contrast injection. The second helical CT scan is initiated as soon as possible after completion of the arterial enhancement phase (interscan delay between 20 and 30 sec). The ideal scanning delay using flow rates < 2 mL/sec has not been established.

Alternatively, a computer automated scanning technology (also referred to as an automated bolus tracking approach) can be used to monitor contrast enhancement and initiate scanning. This technique allows on-line monitoring of contrast enhancement by acquiring very-low-mA scans and region-of-interest measurements at a predetermined level (11). Once an arbitrary threshold level of contrast enhancement has been reached, the series of low-dose scans is terminated and diagnostic scanning is initiated at the top of the scanning volume. This option can be used with either hand or power injections.

By comparison with the abdomen, the initiation of scanning in the chest should begin after 80% of the contrast medium has been administered, regardless of whether contrast is administered by hand or by power injection. Alternatively, scanning can also be initiated with the bolus tracking technique.

In summary, the choice of a protocol for contrast administration in children requires an understanding of contrast dynamics. There is no ideal protocol. Each patient is different and contrast delivery will vary with the route of intravenous access, catheter or needle size, and contrast flow rate.

Bowel Opacification

Bowel opacification is necessary for almost all CT examinations of the abdomen. The exceptions are patients with depressed mental states who are at risk of aspiration and those with acute blunt abdominal trauma where there may be insufficient time for contrast administration. The agent used most often for bowel opacification is a dilute solution of water-soluble iodine-based contrast. The contrast can be given orally or through a nasogastric tube. When administered orally, the contrast may be mixed with Kool-Aid or fruit juice to mask its unpleasant taste.

Contrast material is given 45–60 min before the examination and then again 15 min prior to scanning. The initial volume of oral contrast material should be approximately equal to that of an average feeding. One-half of the total volume is administered 15 min prior to scanning. If adequate opacification of the distal small bowel or colon has not been achieved, additional oral contrast medium can be given and the patient rescanned after a delay to allow the contrast to pass distally. Alternatively, rectal contrast may be administered. The volume of oral contrast material versus patient age is given in Table 2.

IMAGING TECHNIQUES

Helical CT scanning requires optimization of a number of parameters, including scan time duration, table feed speed (the distance to be covered), slice thickness, and reconstruction interval. Generally, in chest and abdominal examinations in older children, 8-mm collimation and 8-mm table speed are used. Decreased collimation (2–4 mm) and decreased table incre-

TABLE 2. *Oral contrast versus age*

Age	Amount given 45 min prior to study	Amount given 15 min prior to scanning
Less than 1 month	2–3 ounces (60–90 mL)	1–1.5 ounces (30–45 mL)
1 month–1 year	4–8 ounces (120–240 mL)	2–4 ounces (60–120 mL)
1–5 years	8–12 ounces (240–360 mL)	4–6 ounces (120–180 mL)
6–12 years	12–16 ounces (360–480 mL)	6–8 ounces (180–240 mL)
13–15 years	16–20 ounces (480–600 mL)	8–10 ounces (240–300 mL)
>15 years	See adult protocols	See adult protocols

ments (2–4 mm) are reserved for very small children, for areas of maximum interest, and for detailed examinations of smaller structures such as pulmonary nodules or the adrenal glands. The table increment is usually set equal to the collimation (pitch = 1), but it may be greater, even doubled relative to collimation (pitch = 2) as long as 180-degree interpolation is used. Scanning with a larger pitch will allow coverage of a greater distance per second of scanning and can be useful in larger patients. However, the disadvantage of an increased pitch is *z*-axis blurring with subsequent degradation of spatial resolution.

CT sections are obtained with breath-holding at suspended inspiration in cooperative patients, usually children over 6 years of age. A single breath-hold technique is recommended over the multiple-breath-hold technique (10–15-sec breath-holds with 10-sec intergroup delays). The advantage of the multiple-breath-holding technique is that it is more easily tolerated, but the disadvantage is the potential for anatomic misregistration between adjacent helical acquisitions. Scans are obtained during quiet respiration in children who cannot cooperate with breath-holding instructions.

Common protocols used for helical CT examinations in children are presented. These protocols provide an approach to the most frequently encountered clinical problems. However, the final imaging approach selected must be individualized for each patient and must address the clinical problem to be answered.

NECK

Applications for helical CT of the neck are (a) differentiation of abscess from lymphadenitis and (b) determination of tumor extent. Typical scan parameters are 4–8-mm slice thickness and 4–8-mm/sec table speed with matching reconstruction intervals. Contiguous axial images usually suffice for diagnosis (Fig. 1).

CHEST

Major applications for helical CT of the chest in children include (a) thoracic survey for metastatic disease; (b) characterization of focal parenchymal masses; (c) assessment of congenital or acquired tracheobronchial tree abnormalities; (d) evaluation of interstitial lung disease; and (e) mediastinal/hilar survey for suspected mass or great vessel anomalies.

Thoracic Survey (Rule Out Pulmonary Nodules)

CT scanning has become the established method for detecting and characterizing pulmonary nodules in children with known malignancies that have a high propensity for pulmonary dissemination. Demonstration of a pulmonary nodule or nodules may lead to additional treatment (surgery, chemotherapy, or radiation). Conventional CT has high sensitivity for identifying pulmonary nodules, but false-negative studies can result from variations in the depth of patient respiration or volume averaging. By enabling contiguous volumetric data acquisition and overlapping reconstructions, helical CT eliminates or minimizes these problems (12–14), even in small children who are scanned during quiet breathing (Fig. 2). The technical parameters for screening surveying the lungs are 4–8-mm slice thickness, 4–8-mm/sec table speed, 1.0 pitch, standard algorithm and 4–8-mm reconstructions. Decreased collimation and table speed should be used in very small children.

Small overlapping reconstructions (2–4 mm) should be used to confirm a nodule suspected on standard images and for instances requiring densitometry. To increase the accuracy of densitometry, the section thickness should be at least one-half of the diameter of the nodule (Fig. 3). Smaller intervals are especially beneficial in nonbreath-holding children.

Focal Mass Characterization

The overlapping volumetric data and multiplanar images created during helical CT are useful to delineate the anatomy of complex congenital lesions (arteriovenous malformations and pulmonary sequestrations) and clarify the relationship of a lesion or nodule to the pleura or to the diaphragm (15). Two- and three-dimensional reconstructions in coronal and sagittal planes are particularly helpful in characterizing a lesion as intraparenchymal or pleural based (Fig. 4). Typical scan parameters for mass characterization include 2–4-mm slice thickness, 2–4-mm/sec table speed, 1.0 pitch, high-resolution algorithm, and reconstruction of overlapping slices every 1 or 2 mm.

Tracheobronchial Tree Assessment

The tracheobronchial tree includes the trachea, carina, mainstem bronchi, and the lobar, segmental, and subsegmental bronchi. These structures are easily definable with helical CT. Common indications prompting CT of the airway are (a) evaluation of congenital anomalies, (b) detection of posttransplantation complications, and (c) identification of bronchiectasis (16–19). By comparison with adults, neoplasia is a rare indication for helical CT of the airway in children. Airway assessment requires a table speed sufficient to allow coverage of the entire trachea and proximal subsegmental bronchi. Typical scan parameters are slice thickness of 2–4 mm, table incrementation of 2–4 mm/sec, 1.0 pitch, and 1–2-mm reconstructions.

The contiguous set of images afforded by helical CT allows identification of virtually all normal segmental bronchi, especially when scans are obtained during suspended inspiration. As a result, detection of congenital anomalies is improved (Fig. 5).

Detection of postoperative complications is improved by the use of multiplanar reconstructions. Small dehiscences and stenoses that are not identifiable on conventional CT can be shown by helical CT (19). The length and width of bronchial stenosis and the size and extent of extraluminal gas are shown best as two- or three-dimensional projections rotated to parallel the long axis of the trachea and bronchi (Fig. 6). Three-dimensional images have the advantage of being viewed as a cine loop, allowing depiction of the entire tracheo-bronchial tree.

Endobronchial tumors are rare in children, but when suspected helical CT offers a noninvasive method for diagnosing tumor and for assessing local extent and invasion. Precise delineation of tumor size and length is important for planning surgical resection. Helical CT, particularly with its multiplanar capabilities, also can be useful in evaluating the central airways for foreign-body aspiration. The foreign body can be precisely localized by helical CT prior to bronchoscopic retrieval.

Interstitial Lung Disease

Indications for CT in interstitial lung disease are (a) determination of extent of known disease prior to biopsy or transplantation, (b) determination of superimposed complications, and (c) determination of unrecognized disease. The advantage of helical CT is faster scan time, which minimizes motion misregistration. A standard examination (4–8-mm collimation and table feed) is performed initially followed by a series of narrow collimation scans (Fig. 7).

Dynamic imaging of the lungs with a rapid series of helical CT scans during forced inhalation and exhalation is a useful adjunct to identify global or focal air-trapping associated with bronchiectasis and small-airway abnormalities, such as bronchiolitis obliterans (Fig. 8). The fast scan times afforded by helical CT allow a comparison of identical levels without motion misregistration (20,21). When diffuse lung disease is suspected, scans are obtained with 1.5–2-mm collimation at three selected levels (the aortic arch, tracheal bifurcation, and lung bases) in forced inspiration and expiration. If focal disease (i.e., bronchiectasis, cystic disease) is suspected on the basis of the screening CT, thinly collimated scans in inspiration and expiration can be limited to the area of abnormality. Specific breathing instructions are given before the scan sequences. Attenuation values are then measured using regions of interest (ROIs) placed in the periphery of the lung. In normal lung, attenuation increases homogeneously during exhalation. In patients with air-trapping there is a paradoxical decrease in lung attenuation with exhalation.

Mediastinal/Hilar Survey

Frequent indications for mediastinal and hilar CT include (a) assessment of blunt thoracic trauma, (b) identification of vascular anomalies, and (c) determination of tumor extent. Axial images provide most of the pertinent information. Multiplanar images are occasionally helpful for clarifying anatomy of vascular lesions. Scan parameters include 4–8-mm slice thickness, 4–8-mm/sec table speed, pitch of 1, standard algorithm, and reconstruction of overlapping slices every 4–8 mm.

CT is the procedure of choice in the evaluation of posttraumatic mediastinal widening suspected or clearly identified on chest radiography. Helical CT studies performed during peak vascular enhancement enable identification of traumatic aneurysms and differentiation between hematoma and mediastinal vascular structures.

A wide range of congenital abnormalities can affect the aorta, superior vena cava, and pulmonary arteries with and without associated cardiac abnormalities. Abnormal position and origin of the great vessels as well as absence and hypoplasia are easily identified with helical CT following administration of intravenous contrast medium (Fig. 9).

The third important indication for helical CT is tumor staging. The reconstruction capabilities of helical CT and more consistent precise delivery of contrast medium improve detection of mediastinal infiltration, vascular occlusion or encasement (Fig. 10), and lymph node enlargement. Helical CT is particularly valuable in detecting smaller nodal masses that otherwise might be missed by conventional CT. The resultant information can facilitate surgical planning or radiation therapy. Finally, helical CT can be used to identify central pulmonary thromboemboli, but this is unlikely to be a frequent problem in children.

ABDOMEN AND PELVIS

Three major categories usually prompt CT examination of the abdomen and pelvis in children: (a) determination of site of origin, extent, and character of an abdominal mass;

(b) determination of the presence or absence of abscess; and (c) evaluation of the extent of injury from blunt abdominal trauma. Less often, CT is used to evaluate parenchymal disease of the liver, kidney, and pancreas, as well as abnormalities of the major abdominal vessels. Typical scan parameters include 8–10-mm slice thickness and table speed with matching reconstructions intervals.

Helical CT has an important role in determining the site of origin and extent of neoplasia. Determination of site of origin is improved by the overlapping reconstruction of volumetric data. Diagnostic confidence about vascular invasion or encasement is increased by imaging during the time of peak vascular opacification. In patients with renal tumors, important information can be obtained by scanning the kidney during early (corticomedullary) and late (collecting system) enhancement (22). Axial images usually suffice for diagnosis and determining tumor extent (Fig. 11). Multiplanar images can be useful as an adjunct to display the relationship of tumor to adjacent vascular or osseous structures (Fig. 12).

CT is the study of choice to confirm the presence of suspected intra-abdominal or pelvic abscess. Increasing the reconstruction frequency of helical CT volumetric data can improve detection of small abscesses and enhance confidence in the diagnosis by demonstrating small gas bubbles (Fig. 13).

Helical CT is particularly well suited for screening patients with trauma who are critically ill. The rapid acquisition of scans helps to minimize the time the patient spends in the CT suite, while scanning during peak vascular enhancement optimizes visualization of parenchymal defects, especially those that signify vascular damage (Figs. 14 and 15).

Pitfalls

Helical CT examinations of the abdomen and pelvis are completed more rapidly than conventional CT examinations, leading to a number of potential pitfalls (23,24). In the spleen, early arterial sinusoidal enhancement produces a heterogeneous appearance that can mimic splenic laceration (see Fig. 14). In the setting of trauma, the absence of a perisplenic hematoma should suggest a flow-related artifact, rather than a laceration or fracture. In the kidney, the cortex enhances before the medulla and collecting system, which can make the diagnosis of medullary and collecting system lesions difficult. Parenchymal abnormalities, such as a striated nephrogram in pyelonephritis or small tumor deposits, as well as traumatic disruptions of the ureteropelvic junction, may be missed on scans performed during early phases of enhancement. Delayed images can minimize these errors. Finally, the helical CT study is often completed before a significant amount of contrast material has been excreted into the bladder. The lack of bladder opacification creates a potential pitfall when pathologic fluid collections are present in the pelvis. Once again, delayed images can help to minimize this potential problem.

SKELETAL SYSTEM

Conventional radiography or scintigraphy remain the studies of choice to detect skeletal abnormalities, but CT can be complementary to these examinations when further definition of an abnormality is required. The major advantages of helical CT in the skeletal system are the fast scan times, which help to decrease motion artifact, and the high-quality two- and three-dimensional reconstructions (25,26). The frequent indications for helical CT of the skeleton in children include (a) characterization of congenital abnormalities in areas of complex anatomy (27), (b) assessment of the extent of complex fractures, and (c) determination of the origin and extent of nidus in osteoid osteoma.

Depending on the lesion size, helical CT is performed with 2–4-mm collimation and 2–4-mm/sec table speed through the area of abnormality. Wider collimation, table speed, and reconstruction intervals are suitable for assessing large joints and bone tumors, whereas narrower collimation, table speed, and reconstruction intervals are necessary for evaluating growth plate fractures and small skeletal lesions and regions of the body (e.g., ankle joint, foot, and wrist).

Developmental hip dysplasia and tarsal coalition are two common congenital anomalies in childhood that are well suited for helical CT. In neonates, developmental dysplasia of the hip is initially assessed with real-time sonography. However, CT is often used to evaluate patients after casting or in cases where the reduction may be unstable. The role of helical CT in dysplasia is assessment of the concentricity of closed reduction. Three-dimensional reconstructions are particularly useful for assessing acetabular coverage and deformity of the femoral head (Fig. 16).

Tarsal coalition is a common cause of rigid flatfoot and peroneal spasm in children. Nearly 70% of tarsal coalitions are talocalcaneal and 30% are calcaneonavicular. Evaluation of suspected tarsal coalition requires that both feet be scanned. Comparison is useful for identifying fibrous or cartilaginous unions, and in addition as many as 50% of talocalcaneal coalitions are bilateral. For talocalcaneal coalitions, scans should be obtained perpendicular to the foot, whereas for calcaneonavicular coalition, scans should parallel the long axis of the foot (Fig. 17). Overlapping axial images are usually diagnostic. Multiplanar reconstructions can provide an additional display of coalition but are not essential for diagnosis.

Helical CT with two- and three-dimensional reconstructions excels in confirming and localizing fractures in areas of complex anatomy, such as those involving the pelvis or ankle. Coronal and sagittal reformations are particularly useful for providing details concerning the integrity of the physeal plate and articular surface, the extent of fragment displacement, and the congruity between osseous structures (Fig. 18). These data are critical in planning surgical or conservative management. In the pelvis, multiplanar reconstructions also help in determining the presence of intra-articular loose bodies.

Although MRI remains the method of choice for evaluating soft tissue and medullary extension of skeletal tumors, helical CT is superior for evaluating matrix calcification, cortical bone involvement, and spatial relationships in complex anatomic sites, such as the pelvis. CT is particularly valuable in localizing the nidus in osteoid osteomas prior to surgical resection. The nidus usually can be identified on routine axial CT scans with narrow collimation, but multiplanar reconstructions are beneficial for displaying the tumor location relative to other bony landmarks (Fig. 19).

REFERENCES

1. Siegel MJ, Luker GD. Pediatric applications of helical (spiral) CT. *Radiol Clin North Am* 1995;33:997–1022.
2. White KS. Invited article: helical/spiral CT scanning: a pediatric radiology perspective. *Pediatr Radiol* 1996; 26:5–14.
3. Bisset GS III, Ball WS. Preparation, sedation, and monitoring of the pediatric patient in the magnetic resonance suite. *Semin Ultrasound CT MR* 1991;12:376–378.
4. Frush DP, Bisset GS III, Hall SC. Pediatric sedation in radiology: the practice of safe sleep. *AJR* 1996;167: 1381–1387.
5. Kaste SC, Young CW. Safe use of power injectors with central and peripheral venous access devices for pediatric CT. *Pediatr Radiol* 1995;26:499–501.
6. Bluemke DA, Fishman EK. Spiral CT of the liver. *AJR* 1993;160:787–792.
7. Heiken JP, Brink JA, Sael SS. Helical CT: abdominal applications. *Radiographics* 1994;14:919–924.
8. Luker GD, Siegel MJ, Bradley DA, Baty JD. Hepatic spiral CT in children: scan delay time-enhancement analysis. *Pediatr Radiol* 1996;26:337–340.
9. Roche KJ, Genieser NB, Ambrosino MM. Pediatric hepatic CT: an injection rate. *Radiology* 1996;26:502–507.

10. Bonaldi VM, Bret PM, Reinhold C, Atri M. Helical CT of the liver: value of an early hepatic arterial phase. *Radiology* 1995;197;357–363.
11. Silverman PM, Roberts S, Tefft MC, et al. Helical CT of the liver: clinical application of an automated computer technique, SmartPrep, for obtaining images with optimal contrast enhancement. *AJR* 1995;165:73–78.
12. Costello P, Anderson W, Blume D. Pulmonary nodule: evaluation with spiral volumetric CT. *Radiology* 1991; 179:875–876.
13. Rémy-Jardin M, Rémy J, Giraud F, Marquette CH. Pulmonary nodules: detection with thick-section spiral CT versus conventional CT. *Radiology* 1993;187:513–520.
14. Wright AR, Collie DA, Williams JR, Hasemi-Malayeri B, Stevenson AJM, Turnbull CM. Pulmonary nodules: effect on detection of spiral CT pitch. *Radiology* 1996;199:837–841.
15. Brink JA, Heiken JP, Semenkovich J, Teefey SA, McClennan BL, Sagel SS. Abnormalities of the diaphragm and adjacent structures; findings on multiplanar spiral CT scans. *AJR* 1994;163:307–310.
16. Kao SC, Smith WL, Franken EA Jr, Kimura K, Soper RT. Ultrafast CT of laryngeal and tracheobronchial obstruction in symptomatic postoperative infants with esophageal atresia and tracheoesophageal fistula. *AJR* 1990;154:345–350.
17. Lucidarme O, Greneir P, Cocke E, Lenoir S, Aubert B, Beigelman C. Bronchiectasis: comparative assessment with thin-section CT and helical CT. *Radiology* 1996;200:673–679.
18. Ney DR, Kuhlman JE, Hruban RH, Ren H, Hutchins GM, Fishman EK. Three-dimensional CT-volumetric reconstruction and display of the bronchial tree. *Invest Radiol* 1990;25:736–742.
19. Quint LE, Whyte RI, Kaserooni EA, et al. Stenosis of the central airways: evaluation by using helical CT with multiplanar reconstructions. *Radiology* 1995;194:871–877.
20. Stern EJ, Webb WR, Golden JA, Gamsu G. Cystic lung disease associated with eosinophilic granuloma and tuberous sclerosis: air-trapping at dynamic ultrafast high-resolution CT. *Radiology* 1992;182:325–329.
21. Stern EJ, Frank MS. Small-airway disease of the lungs: findings at expiratory CT. *AJR* 1994;163:37–41.
22. Zeman RK, Zeiberg A, Hayes WS, Silverman PM, Cooper C, Garra BS. Helical CT of renal masses: the value of delayed scans. *AJR* 1996;167:771–776.
23. Herts BR, Einstein DM, Paushter DM. Spiral CT of the abdomen: artifacts and potential pitfalls. *AJR* 1993; 161:1185–1190.
24. Silverman PM, Cooper CJ, Weltman DI, Zeman RK. Helical CT: practical considerations and potential pitfalls. *Radiographics* 1995;15:225–36.
25. Fishman EK, Magid D, Ney DR, et al. Three-dimensional imaging. *Radiology* 1991;181:321–337.
26. Ney DR, Fishman E, Kawashima A, Robertson D, Scott W. Comparison of spiral CT with serial CT scanning with regard to three-dimensional imaging of musculoskeletal anatomy. *Radiology* 1992;185:865–869.
27. Lee DY, Choi IH, Lee CK, Cho TJ. Assessment of complex hip deformity using three-dimensional CT image. *J Pediatr Orthop* 1991;11:13–19.

Protocol 1: NECK (Fig. 1)

INDICATION:	*Abscess, adenopathy, mass*
SCANNER SETTINGS:	kVp: 120 mAs: 210
PHASE OF RESPIRATION:	Suspended inspiration
SLICE THICKNESS:	4–8 mm
PITCH:	1.0–1.5
SCAN TIME:	Single helical scan: time dependent on patient size
RECONSTRUCTION INTERVAL:	4 mm
SUPERIOR EXTENT:	Base of tongue
INFERIOR EXTENT:	Lung apices

IV CONTRAST:

Concentration:	LOCM 280–320 mg iodine/mL or HOCM 282 mg iodine/mL (60% solution)
Total Volume:	2 mL/kg to maximum of 4 mL/kg (150 mL, maximum)
Rate and Delay:	Determined by method of injection
Hand Injection Rate:	Rapid push bolus
Scan Delay:	Scanning to begin after 80% of bolus given
Power Injector Technique:	Uniphasic injection
Rate:	Dependent on needle size

Rate vs Needle Size

Needle Size	Flow Rate
22 gauge	1.2 mL/sec
20 gauge	1.5 mL/sec
18 gauge	2 mL/sec

Scan Delay:	80% of bolus

COMMENTS:

1. If the child is sedated or uncooperative, CT scans are obtained at quiet breathing.
2. If neck mass is large and easily palpable or if there is clinically significant adenopathy (e.g., lymphomas) 8-mm slice thickness may be adequate as survey.
3. Chest and neck can be examined in a single helical in small children

FIG. 1. Neck masses, contrast enhancement. (**A**) Lymphoma in a 14-year-old boy. Axial CT shows a large nonenhancing, conglomerate mass of nodes (*arrows*) in the right posterior triangle of the neck. The vessels are displaced but patent. (**B**) Thyroid cancer in an 12-year-old boy. Axial CT scan shows an enlarged, heterogeneous left thyroid lobe and an enhancing node (*arrow*) in the left neck.

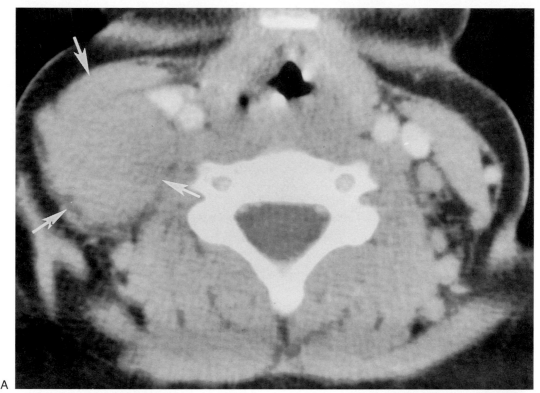

A

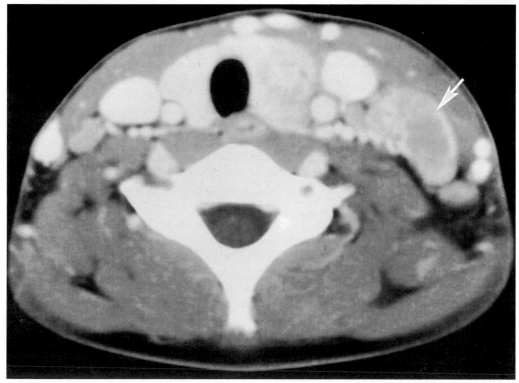

B

Protocol 2:
THORACIC SURVEY (Figs. 2 and 3)

INDICATION:	*Oncologic staging, including metastases, lymphoma*
SCANNER SETTINGS:	kVp: 120 mAs: 210
ORAL CONTRAST:	None
PHASE OF RESPIRATION:	Suspended inspiration
SLICE THICKNESS:	4–8 mm
PITCH:	1.0 up to 1.5
SCAN TIME:	Single helical scan: time dependent on patient size
RECONSTRUCTION INTERVAL:	4–8 mm (contiguous scans)
SUPERIOR EXTENT:	Lung apices
INFERIOR EXTENT:	Caudal lung bases

IV CONTRAST:

Concentration:	LOCM 280–320 mg iodine/mL or HOCM 282 mg iodine/mL (60% solution)
Total Volume:	2 mL/kg to maximum of 4 mL/kg (150 mL, maximum)
Rate and Delay:	Determined by method of injection
Hand Injection Rate:	Rapid push bolus
Scan Delay:	Scanning to begin after 80% of bolus given
Power Injector Technique:	Uniphasic injection
Rate:	Dependent on needle size

Rate vs Needle Size

Needle Size	Flow Rate
22 gauge	1.2 mL/sec
20 gauge	1.5 mL/sec
18 gauge	2 mL/sec

Scan Delay: 80% of bolus

COMMENTS:

1. If the child is sedated or uncooperative, CT scans are obtained at quite breathing.
2. Slice thickness and pitch are dependent on size of the patient; thinner 4-mm contiguous scans and pitch 1.0 can be used in smaller patients.
3. When both chest and abdomen are to be examined, the abdomen should be scanned first. Two-thirds of contrast volume should be given in the abdomen and one-third in the chest.
4. When pulmonary metastases are the chief concern, a noncontrast-enhanced scan may suffice.

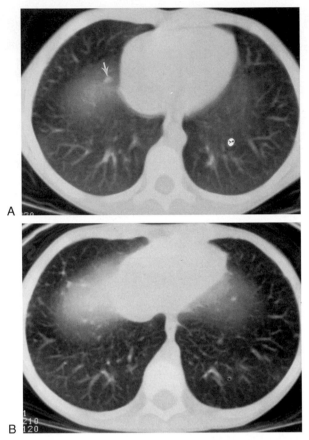

FIG. 2. Pulmonary metastases from thyroid cancer in an 8-year-old boy. (**A**) Section from a conventional CT scan done with 8-mm-thick slices and 8-mm intervals shows a nodule (*arrow*) in the right lower lobe. (**B**) Spiral CT scan, acquired the same day, with 8-mm collimation, 8-mm table feed, and 4-mm reconstruction interval shows several small nodules in the same area.

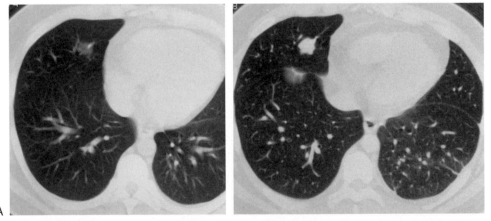

FIG. 3. CT densitometry. (**A**) Axial helical CT scan in a 16-year-old boy with osteogenic sarcoma shows an ill-defined nodule at the right base. (**B**) CT scan reconstructed with 2-mm intervals shows obvious calcification in the mass. Surgical resection confirmed metastatic osteosarcoma.

Protocol 3:
FOCAL PARENCHYMAL MASS (Fig. 4)

INDICATION:	*Tumor, inflammatory, sequestration, and vascular malformation*
SCANNER SETTINGS:	kVp: 120 mAs: 210
ORAL CONTRAST:	None
PHASE OF RESPIRATION:	Suspended inspiration
SLICE THICKNESS:	2–4 mm
PITCH:	1.0
SCAN TIME:	Single helical scan: time dependent on lesion size
RECONSTRUCTION INTERVAL:	1–2 mm
SUPERIOR EXTENT:	Top of area of interest
INFERIOR EXTENT:	Bottom of area of interest

IV CONTRAST:

Concentration:	LOCM 280–320 mg iodine/mL or HOCM 282 mg iodine/mL (60% solution)
Total Volume:	2 mL/kg to maximum of 4 mL/kg (150 mL, maximum)
Rate and Delay:	Determined by method of injection
Hand Injection	
Rate:	Rapid push bolus
Scan Delay:	Scanning to begin after 80% to 100% of bolus given
Power Injector	
Technique:	Uniphasic injection
Rate:	Dependent on needle size

	Rate vs Needle Size	
	Needle Size	**Flow Rate**
	22 gauge	1.2 mL/sec
	20 gauge	1.5 mL/sec
	18 gauge	2 mL/sec
Scan Delay:	100% of contrast medium	

COMMENTS:

1. Slice thickness is dependent on size of lesion; thinner 2-mm scans can be used in smaller patients.
2. Multiplanar reconstructions done with 1-mm or 2-mm interval reconstructions.

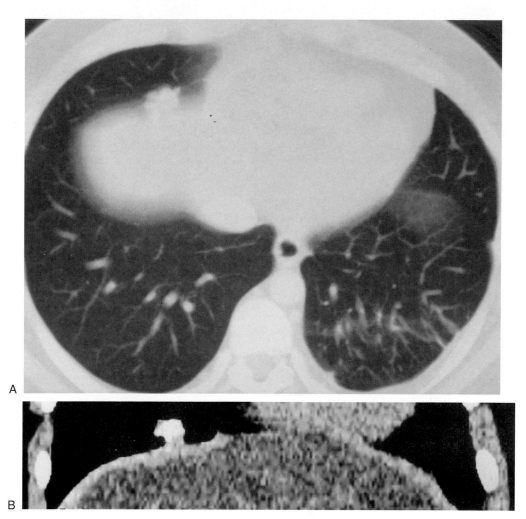

FIG. 4. Peridiaphragmatic metastasis from osteosarcoma in a 14-year-old boy. (**A**) Axial image shows a calcified nodule adjacent to the dome of the liver. The relationship of this mass to the diaphragm was unclear on axial images. (**B**) Sagittal two-dimensional image (4-mm collimation, 2-mm reconstruction) shows that the nodule is in the pulmonary parenchyma but abuts the diaphragm. Open lung exploration confirmed a parenchymal metastasis. (Reprinted with permission from Siegel MJ, Luker GD. Pediatric applications of helical (spiral) CT. *Radiol Clin North Am* 1995;33:997–1022.)

Protocol 4:
TRACHEOBRONCHIAL TREE (Figs. 5 and 6)

INDICATION:	*Congenital anomalies/stenoses/dehiscence*
SCANNER SETTINGS:	kVp: 120 mAs: 210
ORAL CONTRAST:	None
PHASE OF RESPIRATION:	Suspended inspiration
SLICE THICKNESS:	2–4 mm
PITCH:	1.0 up to 1.5
SCAN TIME:	Single helical scan: time dependent on patient size
RECONSTRUCTION INTERVAL:	1–2-mm increments through areas of pathology
SUPERIOR EXTENT:	Top of area of interest
INFERIOR EXTENT:	Bottom of area of interest
IV CONTRAST:	None
COMMENTS:	1. Use high spatial resolution reconstruction (bone) algorithm. 2. Multiplanar reconstructions of the airways require 1-mm or 2-mm interval reconstructions. Used to assess strictures or bronchial dehiscence. 3. Two-dimensional and three-dimensional images provide best airway display.

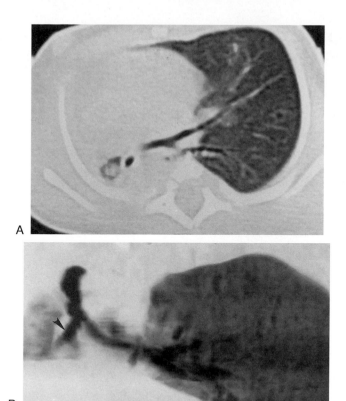

FIG. 5. Hypoplastic lung in a newborn girl. (**A**) Axial shows an opaqued right hemithorax except for a tiny area of aerated lung posteriorly. (**B**) Coronal two-dimensional multiplanar reconstruction (2-mm collimation, 2-mm reconstruction) shows a hypoplastic right mainstem bronchus (*arrowhead*) supplying a small aerated segment of right lung. The remainder of the right hemithorax is opaque because the lung is absent. The left mainstem bronchus and lung are normal.

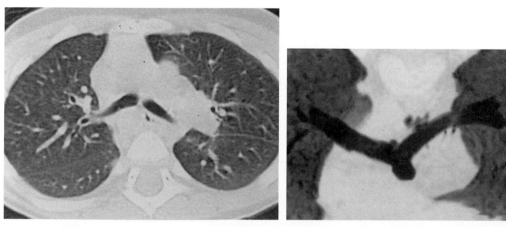

FIG. 6. Bronchial dehiscence in a 3-year-old recipient of a double lung transplant. (**A**) Axial image shows small gas collections (*arrow*) inferior to the left mainstem bronchus. (**B**) Two-dimensional coronal multiplanar image (4-mm collimation, 2-mm reconstruction) shows the gas collections immediately adjacent to the anastomosis of the left mainstem bronchus with the trachea.

Protocol 5:
DIFFUSE LUNG DISEASE (Figs. 7 and 8)

INDICATION:	Extent of interstitial lung disease
SCANNER SETTINGS:	kVp: 120 mAs: 210
ORAL CONTRAST:	None
PHASE OF RESPIRATION:	Suspended inspiration
SLICE THICKNESS:	4–8-mm survey scan; 1.5–2.0-mm thin sections
PITCH:	1.0 for survey scan; second set of scans at 2–3 cm
SCAN TIME:	Single helical scan: time dependent on patient size
RECONSTRUCTION INTERVAL:	4–8 mm for survey scan; 1–2-mm reconstructions for thin section slices
SUPERIOR EXTENT:	Lung apices
INFERIOR EXTENT:	Caudal lung bases
IV CONTRAST:	None
COMMENTS:	1. If the child is sedated or uncooperative, CT scans are obtained at quiet breathing. 2. Initially a survey study of the entire thorax should be performed, using 4–8-mm collimation at 4–8-mm intervals, dependent upon the size of the patient. Then thinner scans using 1.5–2-mm collimation and the high spatial resolution reconstruction (bone) algorithm should be performed every 2–3 cm down to the lung bases when entire lung fields are scanned. 3. Scans can be obtained during forced inhalation and exhalation if air-trapping is a clinical concern

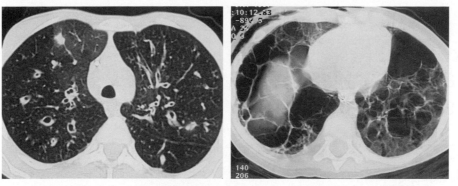

FIG. 7. Interstitial lung diseases. (**A**) Cystic fibrosis in a 8-year-old girl. Axial CT scan at 8-mm thickness and table speed shows hyperinflated lungs with mildly dilated upper lobe bronchi. (**B**) Langerhans cell histiocytosis in a 3-year-old boy. Multiple large, thin-walled cysts are randomly distributed throughout the lungs. Virtually no normal lung tissue is seen.

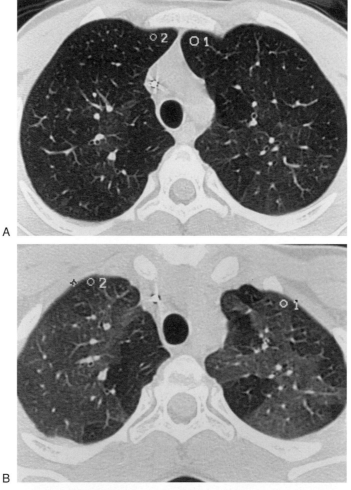

FIG. 8. Dynamic images (2-mm collimation) of the lungs in a 12-year-old boy with a double lung transplant. (**A**) Axial image obtained during full inspiration shows homogeneously aerated lungs. (**B**) Axial image during expiration shows more areas of air-trapping in both upper lobes posteriorly, representing bronchiolitis obliterans (biopsy proven).

Protocol 6: MEDIASTINAL/HILAR SURVEY (Figs. 9 and 10)

INDICATION:	*Trauma, mass lesion, vascular anomaly*
SCANNER SETTINGS:	kVp: 120 mAs: 210
ORAL CONTRAST:	None
PHASE OF RESPIRATION:	Suspended inspiration
SLICE THICKNESS:	4–8 mm
PITCH:	1.0 up to 1.5
SCAN TIME:	Single helical scan: time dependent on patient size.
RECONSTRUCTION INTERVAL:	4–8 mm
SUPERIOR EXTENT:	Lung apices
INFERIOR EXTENT:	Caudal lung bases

IV CONTRAST:

Concentration:	LOCM 280–320 mg iodine/mL or HOCM 282 mg iodine/mL (60% solution)
Total Volume:	2 mL/kg to maximum of 4 mL/kg (150 mL, maximum)
Rate and Delay:	Determined by method of injection
Hand Injection	
Rate:	Rapid push bolus
Scan Delay:	Scanning to begin after 80% of bolus given
Power Injector	
Technique:	Uniphasic injection
Rate:	Dependent on needle size

Rate vs Needle Size

Needle Size	Flow Rate
22 gauge	1.2 mL/sec
20 gauge	1.5 mL/sec
18 gauge	2 mL/sec

Scan Delay:	80% of bolus

COMMENTS:

1. If the child is sedated or uncooperative, CT scans are obtained at quiet breathing.
2. Slice thickness is dependent on size of the patient; thinner 4-mm contiguous scans can be used in smaller patients.

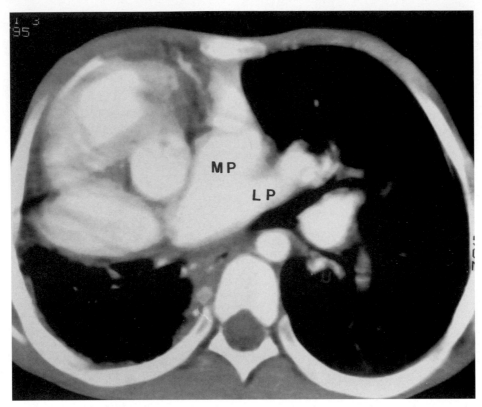

FIG. 9. Hypoplastic right lung and pulmonary artery in a 5-year-old boy. Contrast-enhanced scan at the level of the pulmonary hila demonstrates excellent opacification of the main pulmonary artery (MP) and left pulmonary artery (LP). No pulmonary artery is noted in the right hilum.

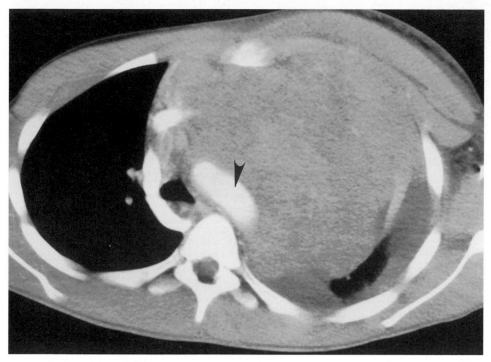

FIG. 10. Lymphoma in a 4-year-old boy. Contrast-enhanced axial CT shows a large anterior mediastinal mass displacing the aortic arch (*arrowhead*) posteriorly. Note absence of visualization of the left brachiocephalic vessel due to compression by tumor. Also noted is a left pleural effusion.

Protocol 7:
ABDOMINAL SURVEY (Figs. 11 and 12)

INDICATION: *Tumor, abscess*

SCANNER SETTINGS: kVp: 120
                           mAs: 210

ORAL CONTRAST: Oral contrast 45 min before scanning. Repeat
                           one-half the amount of oral contrast 15 min
                           prior to scanning.
                           Dose: Determined by patient age.

Dose of Oral Contrast Media Based on Patient Age		
Age	Amount Given 45 Min Prior to Study	Amount Given 15 Min Prior to Scanning
<1 month	2–3 oz (60–90 mL)	1–1.5 oz (30–45 mL)
1 month–1 year	4–8 oz (120–240 mL)	2–4 oz (60–120 mL)
1–5 years	8–12 oz (240–360 mL)	4–6 oz (120–180 mL)
6–12 years	12–16 oz (360–480 mL)	6–8 oz (180–240 mL)
13–15 years	16–20 oz (480–600 mL)	8–10 oz (240–300 mL)
>15 years	See adult protocols	See adult protocols

PHASE OF RESPIRATION: Suspended inspiration

SLICE THICKNESS: 4–8 mm

PITCH: 1.0 up to 1.5

SCAN TIME: Single helical scan: time dependent on patient
                            size.

**RECONSTRUCTION
   INTERVAL:**   4–8 mm

SUPERIOR EXTENT: Diaphragm

INFERIOR EXTENT: Symphysis pubis

IV CONTRAST:

Concentration:	LOCM 280–320 mg iodine/mL or HOCM 282 mg iodine/mL (60% solution)
Total Volume:	2 mL/kg to maximum of 4 mL/kg (150 mL, maximum)
Rate and Delay:	Determined by method of injection
Hand Injection	
Rate:	Rapid push bolus
Scan Delay:	Scanning to begin after 80% to 100% of bolus given
Power Injector	
Technique:	Uniphasic injection
Rate:	Dependent on needle size

Rate vs Needle Size

Needle Size	Flow Rate
22 gauge	1.2 mL/sec
20 gauge	1.5 mL/sec
18 gauge	2 mL/sec

Scan Delay:	100% of contrast

COMMENTS:

1. If the child is sedated or uncooperative, CT scans are obtained at quiet breathing.
2. Slice thickness is dependent on size of patient; thinner 4 mm contiguous scans can be used in smaller patients and for detailed examinations of smaller lesions.

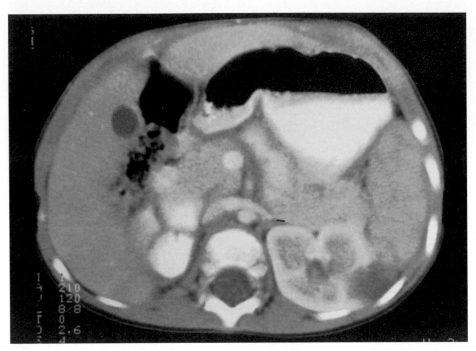

FIG. 11. Wilms tumor. Two-year-old boy status post nephrectomy for right Wilms tumor. Axial image shows no evidence of recurrence in the right renal fossa. A small mass is noted growing exophytically from the left kidney, documented at biopsy to be nephroblastomatosis rather than Wilms tumor.

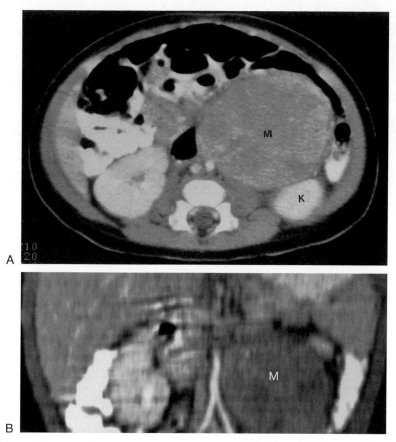

FIG. 12. Neuroblastoma. Two-year-old-boy with left adrenal neuroblastoma. (**A**) Axial image of the abdomen shows a large mass (M) anterior to the left kidney (K). (**B**) Coronal two-dimensional image (4-mm collimation, 4-mm reconstruction interval) displays the size of the mass (M) and its relationship to the aorta. The aorta is not displaced or encased by the mass.

Protocol 8:
PELVIS (Fig. 13)

INDICATION: *Tumor, abscess*

SCANNER SETTINGS: kVp: 120
                             mAs: 210

ORAL CONTRAST: Oral contrast 45 min before scanning. Repeat 1/2
                             of amount 15 min prior to scanning.
                             Dose: Determined by patient age.

Dose of Oral Contrast Media Based on Patient Age		
Age	Amount Given 45 min Prior to Study	Amount Given 15 min Prior to Scanning
<1 month	2–3 oz (60–90 mL)	1–1.5 oz (30–45 mL)
1 month–1 year	4–8 oz (120–240 mL)	2–4 oz (60–120 mL)
1–5 years	8–12 oz (240–360 mL)	4–6 oz (120–180 mL)
6–12 years	12–16 oz (360–480 mL)	6–8 oz (180–240 mL)
13–15 years	16–20 oz (480–600 mL)	8–10 oz (240–300 mL)
>15 years	See adult protocols	See adult protocols

PHASE OF RESPIRATION: Suspended inspiration

SLICE THICKNESS: 4–8 mm

PITCH: 1.0

SCAN TIME: Single helical scan: time dependent on patient
                             size.

**RECONSTRUCTION
  INTERVAL:**   4–8 mm

SUPERIOR EXTENT: Iliac crest

INFERIOR EXTENT: Symphysis pubis

IV CONTRAST:

Concentration:	LOCM 280–320 mg iodine/mL or HOCM 282 mg iodine/mL (60% solution)
Total Volume:	2 mL/kg to maximum of 4 mL/kg (150 mL, maximum)
Rate and Delay:	Determined by method of injection
Hand Injection	
Rate:	Rapid push bolus
Scan Delay:	Scanning to begin after 100% of bolus given
Power Injector	
Technique:	Uniphasic injection
Rate:	Dependent on needle size

Rate vs Needle Size

Needle Size	Flow Rate
22 gauge	1.2 mL/sec
20 gauge	1.5 mL/sec
18 gauge	2 mL/sec

Scan Delay:	100% of contrast injection

COMMENTS:

1. If oral contrast has not reached the colon, a contrast enema may be helpful in defining the rectosigmoid colon. Rectal contrast is not routinely administered.
2. Slice thickness is dependent on size of the patient; thinner 4-mm contiguous scans can be used in smaller patients.

FIG. 13. Pelvic abscesses. (**A**) Crohn's disease in a 12-year-old girl. Axial image demonstrates a small fluid collection with enhanced walls in the right abdominal wall. (**B**) Appendicitis in a 14-year-old boy. Axial image shows a large, well-defined abscess containing air and surrounded by an enhancing wall.

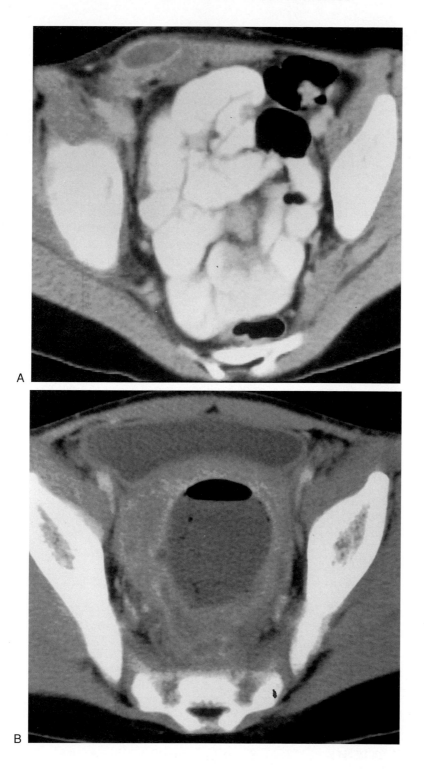

A

B

Protocol 9:
ABDOMINAL TRAUMA SURVEY
(Figs. 14 and 15)

INDICATION:	*Trauma*

SCANNER SETTINGS: kVp: 120
     mAs: 210

ORAL CONTRAST: Water soluble oral contrast 45 min before scanning. Repeat one-half of amount 15 min prior to scanning.

Oral contrast should be used with caution if patient has a depressed level of consciousness, severe injuries, or requires an immediate study.

Dose: Determined by patient age.

Dose of Oral Contrast Media Based on Patient Age		
Age	Amount Given 45 min Prior to Study	Amount Given 15 min Prior to Scanning
<1 month	2–3 oz (60–90 mL)	1–1.5 oz (30–45 mL)
1 month–1 year	4–8 oz (120–240 mL)	2–4 oz (60–120 mL)
1–5 years	8–12 oz (240–360 mL)	4–6 oz (120–180 mL)
6–12 years	12–16 oz (360–480 mL)	6–8 oz (180–240 mL)
13–15 years	16–20 oz (480–600 mL)	8–10 oz (240–300 mL)
>15 years	See adult protocols	See adult protocols

PHASE OF RESPIRATION: Suspended inspiration

SLICE THICKNESS: 4–8 mm

PITCH: 1.0 up to 1.5

SCAN TIME: Single helical scan: time dependent on patient size.

RECONSTRUCTION INTERVAL: 4–8 mm

SUPERIOR EXTENT: Diaphragm

INFERIOR EXTENT: Symphysis pubis

IV CONTRAST:

Concentration:	LOCM 280–320 mg iodine/mL or HOCM 282 mg iodine/mL (60% solution)
Total Volume:	2 mL/kg to maximum of 4 mL/kg (150 mL, maximum)
Rate and Delay:	Determined by method of injection
Hand Injection	
Rate:	Rapid push bolus
Scan Delay:	Scanning to begin after 80% to 100% of bolus given
Power Injector	
Technique:	Uniphasic injection
Rate:	Dependent on needle size

Rate vs Needle Size

Needle Size	Flow Rate
22 gauge	1.2 mL/sec
20 gauge	1.5 mL/sec
18 gauge	2 mL/sec

Scan Delay:	100% of contrast medium

COMMENTS:

1. If amylase is increased or a pancreatic abnormality is suspected, 4-mm-thick scans should be obtained through the pancreas. Pancreatic fractures are often associated with surrounding fluid collections.
2. Need to obtain lung window images to look for pneumothorax and pneumoperitoneum.
3. Slice thickness is dependent on size of the patient; thinner 4-mm contiguous scans can be used in smaller patients.

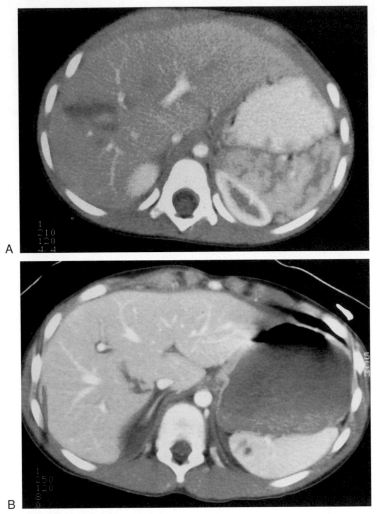

FIG. 14. Hepatic lacerations. (**A**) Axial image obtained during an early arterial phase in a 3-year-old boy shows small, linear lacerations in the right lobe of the liver. Splenic heterogeneity reflects early sinusoidal enhancement. (**B**) Axial image of a 4-year-old boy shows a small laceration medially in the right lobe and small splenic hematomas.

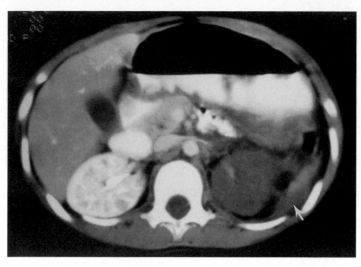

FIG. 15. Vascular pedicle injury. Axial CT scan in a 2-year-old boy shows a nonenhancing left kidney caused by avulsion of the renal pedicle. Fluid is also noted in the lateral conal fascia (arrow).

Protocol 10:
HIPS (Fig. 16)

INDICATION:	*Evaluate acetabular/femoral congruity*
SCANNER SETTINGS:	kVp: 120 mAs: 210
ORAL CONTRAST:	None
PHASE OF RESPIRATION:	Quiet breathing
SLICE THICKNESS:	2–4 mm
PITCH:	1.0
SCAN TIME:	Single helical scan: time dependent on patient size.
RECONSTRUCTION INTERVAL:	2 or 4 mm
SUPERIOR EXTENT:	Acetabular roof
INFERIOR EXTENT:	Femoral necks
IV CONTRAST:	None
COMMENTS:	1. Slice collimation is dependent on size of patient. 2. Two- and three-dimensional reconstructions should be routinely obtained.

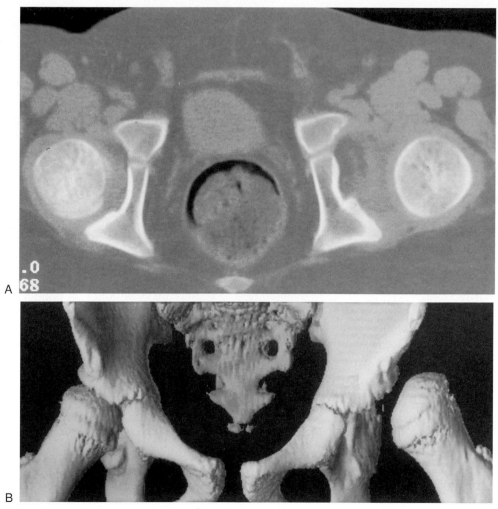

FIG. 16. Developmental hip dysplasia in an 2-year-old boy. (**A**) Axial image shows a laterally displaced left femoral head. The right femoral head is normally seated. (**B**) Coronal image (4-mm collimation, 2-mm reconstruction) displays superior and lateral dislocation of the left femur and a dysplastic acetabulum.

Protocol 11:
TARSAL COALITION (Fig. 17)

INDICATION:	*Congenital*
SCANNER SETTINGS:	kVp: 120 mAs: 210
ORAL CONTRAST:	None
PHASE OF RESPIRATION:	Quiet breathing
SLICE THICKNESS:	2 mm
PITCH:	1.0
SCAN TIME:	Single helical scan: time dependent on patient size
RECONSTRUCTION INTERVAL:	1 or 2 mm
SUPERIOR EXTENT:	Begin just anterior to talus
INFERIOR EXTENT:	Through mid-calcaneus past talocalcaneal joint
IV CONTRAST:	None
COMMENTS:	1. For talocalcaneal coalition, the ideal imaging position is with the patient supine, knees flexed, and feet flat on the gantry table. Tape the feet to the gantry table to prevent inadvertent motion. 2. For suspected calcaneonavicular coalition, the patient is positioned with legs extended and feet and toes vertical to the table. 3. Scans routinely obtained with bone algorithm.

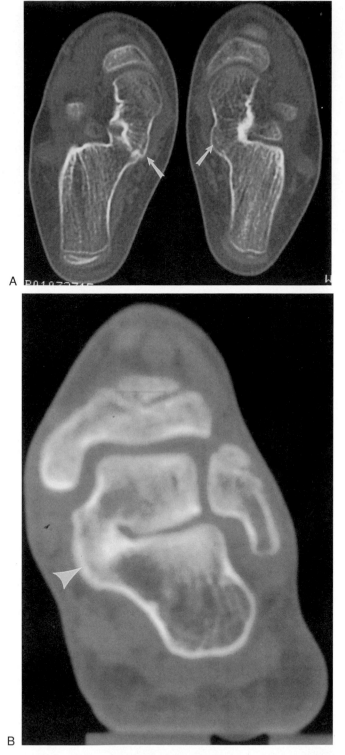

FIG. 17. Tarsal coalitions. (**A**) Scan in a 12-year-old boy through the long axis of the hindfeet shows bilateral calcaneonavicular coalitions (*arrows*). (**B**) Short-axis scan in a 12-year-old boy shows a bony coalition of the talocalcaneal joint (*arrowhead*).

Protocol 12:
LOCALIZED BONE LESION
(Figs. 18 and 19)

INDICATION:	*Osteoid osteoma, complex fracture*
SCANNER SETTINGS:	kVp: 120 mAs: 210
ORAL CONTRAST:	None
PHASE OF RESPIRATION:	Quiet breathing
SLICE THICKNESS:	2 mm
PITCH:	1.0
SCAN TIME:	Single helical scan: time dependent on patient size.
RECONSTRUCTION INTERVAL:	1–2 mm
SUPERIOR EXTENT:	Superior extent of abnormality identified on topogram
INFERIOR EXTENT:	Inferior extent of abnormality identified on topogram
IV CONTRAST:	None
COMMENTS:	1. Collimation and table speed dependent on lesion size. 2. Use high-resolution algorithm for reconstruction.

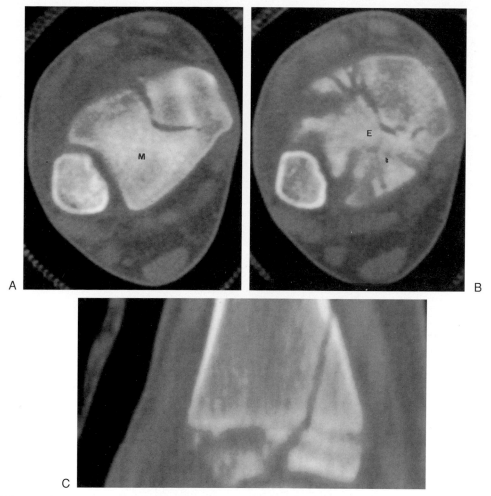

FIG. 18. Triplane fracture in a 12-year-old girl. (**A**) and (**B**) two axial CT images show fractures of the metaphysis (M) and epiphysis (E) of the right ankle. (**C**) Sagittal multiplanar image (2-mm collimation, 2-mm reconstruction) shows the vertical component of the fracture, but it also shows step-off in the articular surface, requiring open fixation.

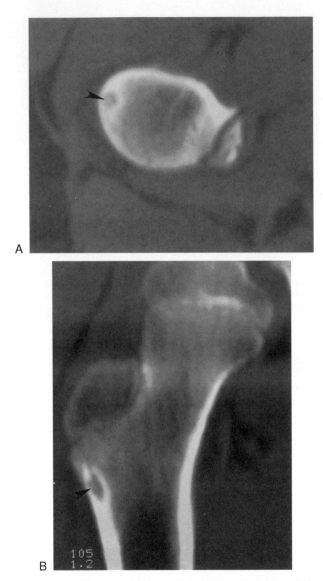

FIG. 19. Osteoid osteoma in a 13-year-old boy. (**A**) Axial image shows a lytic nidus (*arrowhead*) with faint calcification in the lateral cortex of the proximal right femur. The cortex around the nidus is thickened. (**B**) Coronal reconstruction image demonstrates the nidus (*arrowhead*) and its relationship to the greater trochanter. (Reprinted with permission from Siegel MJ, Luker GD. Pediatric applications of helical [spiral] CT. *Radiol Clin North Am* 1995;33:997–1022.)

Helical (Spiral) Computed Tomography,
edited by Paul M. Silverman.
Lippincott–Raven Publishers, Philadelphia © 1998.

7

Protocols for Helical CT for Three-Dimensional Imaging

Geoffrey D. Rubin

*Department of Radiology, Stanford University School of Medicine,
Stanford, California 94305*

Because helical computed tomography (CT) data are volumetric, they are well suited to three-dimensional visualization (1). However, the quality of three-dimensional images is highly dependent on the quality of the acquired CT data. The use of three-dimensional rendering must be anticipated prior to image acquisition, to optimize the data available for rendering. This section first reviews relevant acquisition, contrast administration, and reconstruction issues for optimizing three-dimensional visualization of the blood vessels, airways, and colon; then the most commonly available rendering techniques and tools for prerendering data preparation (editing) are discussed.

ACQUISITION OPTIMIZATION

The two fundamental determinants of the acquisition parameters are anatomic coverage and acquisition time. The anatomic coverage is dictated by the craniocaudal extent of the relevant anatomy, which in turn determines the table travel distance. In the chest and abdomen the acquisition time is typically determined by breath-hold duration. Outside of these regions, where ventilatory misregistration occurs, the primary limitation to the acquisition time is the patient's tolerance for iodinated contrast, as longer scans require more contrast.

The Table Speed is thus determined as Anatomic Coverage (mm) divided by Acquisition Duration (sec). Once the table speed is determined, then the collimation can be calculated as Table Speed divided by Pitch. To complete this calculation two additional parameters must be known: gantry rotation time and pitch. The gantry rotation time should be selected as the shortest time available, typically 0.75–1.0 sec. To select the pitch we must review some information. We know that the effective section thickness (full width at half maximum of the section sensitivity profile) is broadened by 30% when pitch is increased from 1.0 to 2.0 and data are reconstructed with 180-degree linear interpolation (2,3). We also know that when data are reconstructed with 360-degree linear interpolation, the effective section thickness is 30% broader at pitch 1.0 than the same data reconstructed with 180-degree interpolation and that the effective section thickness increases by 116% when pitch is increased to 2.0 (2). Therefore when optimizing the longitudinal resolution of any helical CT acquisition, 180-degree linear interpolation should be used over 360-degree interpolation. Furthermore, in general, pitch should be a value close to 2.0 that allows the calculation of the collimation to provide a width that is available on the scanner (i.e., whole numbers 1, 2, 3, 5, . . .) (4). This may not be immediately intuitive, so let us consider an example by defining two scan protocols designed to cover the same anatomic coverage (15 cm) during the same acquisition duration (30 sec). The table speed will thus be the same for both acquisitions (5 mm/sec), so we have a choice of 5-mm collimation, pitch 1.0 versus 3-mm collimation, pitch 1.7. The effective section thickness of the former is 5 mm, whereas the effective section thickness of the latter is 3.6 mm, using 180-degree linear interpolation. Therefore using a scan protocol with a higher pitch (1.7 vs. 1.0) allows us to narrow the collimation (3 vs. 5 mm) and improve the longitudinal spatial resolution by 28%.

CONTRAST ADMINISTRATION

A critical factor that determines the quality of three-dimensional renderings is the contrast-to-noise ratio. Therefore for any CT application where three-dimensional visualization is desired, the contrast differential between the structures of interest and the background tissues should be maximized. Although this does not present difficulties for airway or colonic visualization, where gas provides naturally high contrast, in the blood vessels contrast opacification must be maximized with intravascular contrast medium. Iodinated contrast media are administered through an antecubital vein. To ensure maximal vascular opacification, a tight bolus is delivered such that the bolus duration is equivalent to the scan duration (i.e., a 40-sec-long helical scan requires a 40-sec-long bolus). As a result, the contrast dosage and flow rate are related as follows:

1. Contrast Medium Volume (mL)

$$= \text{Contrast Medium Flow Rate (mL/sec)} \times \text{Scan Duration(s)}$$

or

2. Contrast Medium Flow Rate (mL/sec)

$$= \text{Contrast Medium Volume (mL)} \div \text{Scan Duration(s)}$$

In general, contrast medium with at least 300 mg I/mL injected at a flow rate of 4 mL/sec is required to achieve consistent opacification within the adult arterial system for high-quality three-dimensional visualization. This value can be reduced to 3–3.5 mL/sec in patients weighing less than 60 kg. For patients weighing more than 120 kg, higher flow rates may be required. Unless a compelling reason exists to limit the iodinated contrast dosage, such as azotemia, the volume of contrast that allows contrast delivery at the appropriate flow rate for a period equivalent to the scan duration should be administered. If contrast dosage must be limited, then the maximum tolerable volume of contrast should be established and the flow rate and/or scan duration should be modified accordingly (see equation 2 above).

Prior to initiating computed tomographic angiography (CTA), one additional variable must be measured for optimizing the contrast delivery, the scan delay time. Because the bolus duration is equivalent to the scan duration, the enhancement plateau in the arteries of interest must coincide perfectly with the helical CT acquisition. To achieve this, the circulation time for contrast to travel from the site of injection to the target anatomy must be determined individually. Although a delay time of 16–24 sec prior to scan initiation will likely work in 75% of adults and 95% of adults below 50 years of age, the majority of CTA is performed in patients over 50 years who have coexistent vascular disease, frequently involving the heart. As a result, it can be impossible to predict the appropriate scan delay time without a preliminary test injection of contrast material. This is performed with 10–15 mL of contrast medium, injected at a rate of 4 mL/sec. After an 8-sec delay, 5–10-mm transverse sections are acquired every 2–3 sec at the anticipated initiation site of the CTA until 40–45 sec have elapsed since the bolus began. A time–density curve is created by positioning a region of interest (ROI) within the center of the vessel. The peak of the curve is selected as the delay time between bolus initiation and scan initiation (5).

RECONSTRUCTION

As mentioned earlier, the quality of three-dimensional renderings depends on the contrast-to-noise ratio of the cross sections. Therefore a low-noise reconstruction kernel should be used (i.e., soft or standard, not sharp or bone). Additionally, the field of view should be limited to include the anatomy of interest, rather than subcutaneous tissues. This approach improves the in-plane resolution substantially. Typical in-plane fields of view should be 18–25 cm rather than 36–40 cm, as is the case for many routine adult chest, abdomen, or pelvic scans. One cautionary note, however, is that many workstations will only render a longitudinal dimension that is less than or equal to the transverse field of view. Therefore if the table travel distance (anatomic coverage) is greater than the reconstructed field of view, then portions of the data will be cut off from a three-dimensional view oriented to visualize the longitudinal axis. If a single three-dimensional view that displays all the imaged anatomy is desired, then a practical rule is to reconstruct the data with a field of view that is equivalent to the table travel distance.

One additional critical element for reconstructing the data is that overlapping cross sections should always be generated at a frequency that is at least 50% of the collimator width. This improves the longitudinal spatial resolution of the scan and substantially improves the quality of three-dimensional renderings (6).

RENDERING

Four main visualization techniques are currently in use on clinical three-dimensional workstations: multiplanar reformation (MPR), maximum-intensity projections (MIP), shaded-surface renderings (SR), and volume rendering (VR). The first two techniques are limited to external visualization; the latter two allow for immersive or internal visualization and can be used for endoscopic-type applications.

MPR is a very convenient and available technique for displaying the data. One substantial limitation of traditional MPR is that visualized structures must lie in a plane. Because almost all structures for which three-dimensional visualization is desired do not lie within a single plane, an MPR cannot be created that demonstrates the entirety of a structure. As structures course in and out of the MPR, pseudostenoses are created. The solution to this problem is to use curved planar reformations (CPR). Similar to MPR, CPR is a single-voxel-thick tomogram, but it is capable of demonstrating an uninterrupted longitudinal cross section because the display plane curves along the structure of interest. CPRs are created from points that are manually positioned over a structure of interest as viewed on transverse sections, MPRs, MIPs, SRs, or VRs. The points are connected to form a three-dimensional curve that is then extruded through the volume perpendicular to the desired view to create the CPR. CPRs are very useful for displaying the interior of tubular structures, such as blood vessels, airways, and bowel. They are also useful for visualizing structures immediately adjacent to these lumena, such as mural thrombus and extrinsic or exophytic neoplasia, without any editing of the data. An important limitation of CPRs is that they are highly dependent on the accuracy of the curve. Inaccurately positioned or insufficient numbers of points can result in the curve slipping off the structure of interest, creating pseudostenoses. Further, a single curve cannot adequately display eccentric lesions; therefore two curves that are orthogonal to each other should always be created two provide a more complete depiction of eccentric lesions, particularly stenoses.

MIPs are created when a specific projection is selected (anteroposterior, for example); then rays are cast perpendicular to the view through the volume data, with the maximum value encountered by each ray encoded on a two-dimensional output image (7,8). As a result, the entire volume is collapsed, with only the brightest structures visible. Variations of this approach include the minimum-intensity projection (MinIP), which can be useful for visualizing airways (9), and the raysum or average projection (10), which sums all pixel values encountered by each ray to provide an image similar to a radiograph.

An advantage of MIPs over MPRs is that structures that do not lie in a single plane are visible in their entirety. A limitation of MIPs, however, is that bones or other structures that are more attenuative than contrast-enhanced blood vessels, for example, will obscure the blood vessels. Similarly, when creating MinIPs, air external to the patient will obscure the airways and surrounding lung. There are two approaches to addressing these limitations: slab-MIP and prerendering editing. Slab-MIPs are created when a plane through the data is defined and then thickened perpendicular to the plane (11). The process with which the plane is thickened can be MIP, MinIP, raysum, or VR. By selecting a slab orientation that does not result in overlap, extremely high-attenuation structures (bones or metal) and structures of interest (blood vessels), the structures of interest can be clearly visualized without the need for time-consuming and operator-dependent editing. This approach, however, is generally limited to allowing visualization through slabs that are 5–30 mm thick. If a MIP of a larger subvolume of the scan data is desired, then the data typically must be edited to remove obscuring structures. The techniques for editing are discussed in the subsequent section. Even after the issues of obscuration are addressed, MIPs have a couple of lingering limitations. They do not provide for an appreciation of depth relationships, and in regions of complex anatomy, such as at the neck of an aortic aneurysm, it can be difficult to be confident when the true origin of a branch is visualized versus a foreshortened branch caused by overlap of its proximal extent with the aorta itself.

Shaded-surface renderings provide exquisite three-dimensional representations of anatomy, relying on gray scale to encode surface reflections from an imaginary source of illumination (12,13). The majority of SRs created on clinical workstations display a single surface that is the interface between user-selected thresholds. As a result, the 12-bit CT data are reduced to binary data, with each pixel being either within or outside of the threshold range. Some workstations allow several threshold ranges to be defined and displayed with different-colored surfaces. In this setting different tissue types or structures are coded as different colors to facilitate their visualization relative to adjacent structures. For each classification, data segmentation is required, typically by both thresholding and editing, which increases the required processing time arithmetically. Regardless of the number of tissue groups or classes assigned, the selection of the threshold range that defines each class is typically arbitrary and can substantially limit the accuracy of data interpretation, particularly when attempting to grade stenoses. This is particularly true when calcified plaque accompanies regions of arterial stenosis. The plaque typically falls within the same threshold range as blood vessel lumen, resulting in the spurious appearance of a local dilation, rather than a stenosis (14).

The final and most complex rendering technique is VR (15–19). There are many different versions and interfaces for VR, but the general approach is that all voxel values are assigned an opacity level that varies from total transparency to total opacity. This opacity function can be applied to the histogram of voxel values as a whole or to regions of the histogram that are classified as specific tissue types. With the latter approach, rectangular or trapezoidal regions areas are selected that correspond to the range of attenuation values for a structure

(20,21). The walls of the trapezoid slope from an opacity plateau to the baseline of complete transparency in an attempt to account for partial volume effects at the edges of structures. Regions at the walls of the trapezoidal regions or in positions where the opacity curve has a steep slope are referred to as *transition zones* in the ensuing protocols and are analogous to threshold levels with SRs. Lighting effects may be simulated in a fashion similar to that with SR. Because there is no surface definition with VR, lighting effects are applied based upon the spatial gradient (i.e., variability of attenuation within a local neighborhood of voxels). Near the edges of structures, the spatial variation in attenuation changes more rapidly (a high gradient) than in the center of structures (a low gradient). Lighting effects are most pronounced in regions of high spatial gradients. Because lighting effects and variations in transparency are simultaneously displayed, it is frequently useful to view VRs in color. The color is applied to the attenuation histogram to allow differentiation of voxel values and to avoid ambiguity with lighting effects, which are encoded in gray scale. Other variables such as specular reflectivity, which models the shininess of a surface, may be available but should be used with caution to avoid confounding the visualization.

EDITING

The challenge of performing efficient and accurate three-dimensional visualization of clinical CT data is to balance the use of visualization techniques that require editing versus those that do not. In general, it is preferable to avoid time-consuming editing; however, this is unavoidable on most clinical workstations in 1997. Editing can span from very quick and simple interactive cut-plane selection to meticulous two-dimensional ROI selection, with intermediate steps being provided by three-dimensional ROI editing, region growing or connectivity, and slab editing.

When viewing SRs or VRs, the use of cut-planes can be very helpful to remove obscuring structures that lie between our viewpoint and the anatomy of interest. Cut-planes can usually be oriented arbitrarily, but for the same reasons that MPRs are limited for visualizing curved structures, cut-planes are limited for removing curved structures.

A three-dimensional ROI edit is performed when a ROI is selected by drawing a rectangle or more complex shape and extruding this shape through the volume along an appropriate linear path. The selected region is either removed or exclusively retained for rendering. This is a very quick technique that requires the drawing of a single ROI that can then be applied to many cross sections. It can be useful for eliminating the air around the chest when creating MinIPs or for removing the spine from data sets containing only the cervical or lumbar regions of the spine. The easiest way to implement this type of edit is to create a MIP from above or below that allows a cleavage plane to be identified between the spine and the aorta, for example. This usually requires a 10–20-degree anterior rotation of the superior aspect of the volume to correct for lumbar lordosis. Unfortunately, this type of editing is insufficient for removing the pelvis, skull, or large portions of the rib cage, particularly near the thoracic inlet, where a cleavage plane between anatomy of interest and obscuring structures cannot be identified.

There are two main approaches for dealing with this problem: region-growing/connectivity and slab editing. Both can be very effective, but in general region growing is the most flexible and efficient when combined with Boolean operations, such as subtraction. Region growing or connectivity is a threshold-based process, where a seed point is selected in the structure of interest and allowed to grow into contiguous pixels that are within a defined threshold range. Region growing is rarely adequate as the sole editing tool, because there are typically regions of leakage where the seed may grow into undesirable structures. To combat this problem, limited cut-planes or scalpel cuts can be applied over a variable number of sections to disconnect the structures. A typical application of this technique is the disconnection of the superior gluteal arteries from the sacrum as they exit the pelvis. These predictable sites of leakage between the arteries and bones can be disconnected in seconds. A quick search of the remainder of the cross sections may reveal problematic osteophytes contacting the aorta, which must be similarly disconnected; then the region growing is applied and the aorta and its branches can be selected. There are two approaches to using region growing for editing CT data. The first and most intuitive is the selection of the structure of interest and deletion of all unselected pixels from the data. This approach has several limitations. First, the structure of interest may not be identifiable with a single region growing step, such as both sides of an occluded blood vessel reconstituted distally by collateral flow or a highly stenotic vessel that becomes discontinuous with thresholding. Second, the edges of structures will be arbitrarily truncated at the threshold selected for the region growing. Therefore the edge pixels that represent a partial volume effect mediated transition between the structure of interest and the background are excluded. Although SRs will look fine, MIPs will appear as if they have been cut from the data with scissors. This latter limitation can be combated with a simple dilation step, where the editing is allowed to relax by one to four pixels to include these edges; however, the former limitation cannot be addressed by dilation. As a result, the preferred approach is to use region growing to identify the bones, dilate them by three or four pixels to include the edges, and subtract them from the original data. A MIP of 200 abdomen and pelvis transverse sections can be edited in less than 5 min using this approach to display the aortoiliac system free of overlapping bones. The edited data can also be used to create SRs free of bones, providing a posterior view of the aorta and its branches.

Slab editors can also provide an efficient means of editing the data. Slab editors work by allowing the user to preselect variable-thickness slabs of data. The slabs are displayed as slab-MIPs, and a ROI is drawn on each slab. Fewer slabs require less ROI drawing, but more slabs may be required to remove complex structures. For many applications, five to 10 transverse sections are used per slab, improving the efficiency over two-dimensional ROI editing by a factor of 5–10. This technique can be limited in regions such as the pelvis, where the iliac arteries lie close to the pelvic sidewall and the pelvis has a sloping contour, or at the skull base adjacent to the circle of Willis.

The most time-consuming editing technique is section-by-section two-dimensional ROI, where an ROI is drawn individually on each cross section. This provides the most control but is extremely time-consuming and should be reserved only for situations where none of the preceding approaches suffices.

ENDOLUMINAL VISUALIZATION

The ability of helical CT to image the inner surfaces of tubular lumena has led to proposed clinical applications of virtual endoscopy to examine the bowel (19,22,23), airways (19,24–26), blood vessels (19,27), and urinary tract (28,29). Although very little clinical validation of the utility of these techniques exist, they have generated considerable interest among radiologists and other clinicians. Although the term *virtual endoscopy* is catchy, it is vague and applies loosely to any technique that displays the interior of tubular lumena.

The interior surface of tubular lumena can be visualized with SR or VR. The basic approach is to identify threshold levels for SR that exclude pixels of similar attenuation to the lumen (-900 to -1000 HU for air-filled lumena and 150–400 HU for contrast-enhanced blood vessels) or an opacity curve for VR that results in complete transparency of the lumen. It is important to recognize that these renderings allow visualization of the interface between luminal contrast and extraluminal attenuation, not the mucosal or intimal surface. Once the intraluminal pixels have been eliminated or rendered transparent, a view must be created that allows unobstructed intraluminal visualization. Toward that end, two main strategies can be employed: orthographic external rendering with cut-planes and immersive perspective rendering.

Orthographic renderings are the most common type of rendering, particularly for external visualization, and are based upon the assumption that light rays reaching our eyes are parallel, as if structures were viewed with a high-powered telescope from far away. As a result, the proximity of structures to the viewpoint does not influence the size with which they are rendered. This approach is contrasted to perspective rendering below. Although orthographic rendering is exclusively used for visualization from a viewpoint that is external to the data, it can be used for internal visualization when combined with cut-planes that are positioned within the lumen of the structure of interest. This is analogous to cutting a window into a piece of pipe to visualize its interior. This technique is mostly useful for providing regional snapshots, but currently cannot provide a continuous display of all interior surfaces within a tubular lumen. Greater inner-surface visualization is available with immersive rendering.

Immersive rendering implies that the viewpoint is within the data set. To understand depth relationships from close range, structures must be viewed with perspective, which is a modeling that demonstrates spatial relationships similar to the human visual system, where light rays are focused to converge on the retina. The phenomenon of perspective helps us recognize the distance of structures based upon their size, as a structure close to the eye appears larger than a structure further away. The extent to which this effect is observed is determined by the FOV of our virtual lens, which is typically defined as the size of the angle at the apex of a cone of visualization emanating from our viewpoint. A larger angle indicates greater perspective and thus greater disparity in size–distance relationships. Most perspective renderings of CT data are created with a 20–90-degree FOV. Both SRs and VRs can be rendered with perspective and used to create endoluminal views that mimic fiberoptic endoscopy without the mechanical limitations of access to the lumen and view direction. The greatest challenge of immersive visualization is navigation. Flying a virtual endoscope is akin to flying a helicopter. There are three spatial degrees of freedom for position and three spatial degrees of freedom for view direction. When considered with the challenge of appropriate threshold (SR) or opacity table (VR) selection and color, the complexity of creating these visualizations can be daunting. Further, without some external indication of the view position, either on a three-dimensional model or on MPRs, it is easy to lose track of one's location within the lumen. Techniques that automatically create a flight path through the center of a lumen are being developed and are showing promising results. Many variations on the performance of virtual endoscopy, aimed at improving efficiency and ease, will probably be developed in the near future. However, until these techniques are validated against an established standard, CT endoscopy will remain predominantly a research tool.

REFERENCES

1. Rubin GD, Napel S, Leung A. Volumetric analysis of volume data: achieving a paradigm shift. *Radiology* 1996; 200:312–317.
2. Polacin A, Kalender WA, Marchal G. Evaluation of section sensitivity profiles and image noise in spiral CT. *Radiology* 1992;185:29–35.
3. Kasales CJ, Hopper KD, Ariola DN, et al. Reconstructed helical CT scans: improvement in z-axis resolution compared with overlapped and nonoverlapped conventional CT scans. *AJR* 1995;164:1281–1284.
4. Rubin GD, Napel S. Increased scan pitch for vascular and thoracic spiral CT. *Radiology* 1995;197:316–317.
5. Rubin GD. Spiral (helical) CT of the renal vasculature. *Semin Ultrasound CT MRI* 1996;17:374–397.

6. Kalender WA, Polacin A, Süss C. A comparison of conventional and spiral CT: an experimental study on the detection of spherical lesions. *J Comput Assist Tomogr* 1994;18:167–176.
7. Keller PJ, Drayer BP, Fram EK, Williams KD, Dumoulin CL, Souza SP. MR angiography with two-dimensional acquisition and three-dimensional display. *Radiology* 1989;173:527–532.
8. Napel S, Bergin CJ, Paranjpe DV, Rubin GD. Maximum and minimum intensity projection of spiral CT data for simultaneous 3D imaging of the pulmonary vasculature and airways (abstr). *Radiology* 1992;185(P):126.
9. Rubin GD. Techniques of reconstruction. In: M. Rémy-Jardin and J. Rémy, eds., *Spiral CT of the chest.* Berlin: Springer-Verlag, 1996;101–128.
10. Zeman RK, Berman PM, Silverman PM, Davros WJ, Cooper C, Kladakis AO, Gomes MN. Diagnosis of aortic dissection: value of helical CT with multiplanar reformation and three-dimensional rendering. *AJR* 1995;164: 1375–1380.
11. Napel S, Rubin GD, Jeffrey Jr RB. STS-MIP: a new reconstruction technique for CT of the chest. *J Comput Assist Tomogr* 1993;17:832–838.
12. Cline HE, Lorensen WE, Souza SP, et al. 3D surface rendered MR images of the brain and its vasculature. *J Comput Assist Tomogr* 1991;15:344–351.
13. Magnusson M, Lenz R, Danielsson PE. Evaluation of methods for shaded surface display of CT volumes. *Comput Med Imaging Graph* 1991;15:247–256.
14. Rubin GD, Dake MD, Napel S, et al. Spiral CT of renal artery stenosis: comparison of three-dimensional rendering techniques. *Radiology* 1994;190:181–189.
15. Drebin RA, Carpenter L, Hanrahan P. Volume rendering. *Comput Graphics* 1988;22:65–74.
16. Levoy M. Methods for improving the efficiency and versatility of volume rendering. *Prog Clin Biol Res* 1991; 363:473–488.
17. Rusinek H, Mourino MR, Firooznia H, Weinreb JC, Chase NE. Volumetric rendering of MR images. *Radiology* 1989;171:269–272.
18. Fishman EK, Drebin B, Magid D, et al. Volumetric rendering techniques: applications for three-dimensional imaging of the hip. *Radiology* 1987;163:737–738.
19. Rubin GD, Beaulieu CF, Argiro V, et al. Perspective volume rendering of CT and MR images: applications for endoscopic imaging. *Radiology* 1996;199:321–330.
20. Johnson PT, Heath DG, Bliss DF, Cabral B, Fishman EK. Three-dimensional CT: real-time interactive volume rendering. *AJR* 1996;167:581–583.
21. Kuszyk BS, Heath DG, Bliss DF, Fishman EK. Skeletal 3-D CT: advantages of volume rendering over surface rendering. *Skeletal Radiol* 1996;25:207–214.
22. Hara AK, Johnson CD, Reed JE, Ehman RL, Ilstrup DM. Colorectal polyp detection with CT colography: two-versus three-dimensional techniques. Work in progress [see comments]. *Radiology* 1996;200:49–54.
23. Hara AK, Johnson CD, Reed JE, et al. Detection of colorectal polyps by computed tomographic colography: feasibility of a novel technique. *Gastroenterology* 1996;110:284–290.
24. Ferretti GR, Vining DJ, Knoplioch J, Coulomb M. Tracheobronchial tree: three-dimensional spiral CT with bronchoscopic perspective. *J Comput Assist Tomogr* 1996;20:777–781.
25. Vining DJ, Liu K, Choplin RH, Haponik EF, Fishman EK. Virtual bronchoscopy: relationships of virtual reality endobronchial simulations to actual bronchoscopic findings. *Chest* 1996;109:549–553.
26. Naidich DP, Grudrn JF, McGuinness G, McCauley DI, Bhalla M. Volumetric (helical/spiral) CT (VCT) of the airways. *J Thorac Imag* 1997;12:11–28.
27. Kimura F, Shen Y, Date S, Azemoto S, Mochizuki T. Thoracic aortic aneurysm and aortic dissection: new endoscopic mode for three-dimensional CT display of aorta. *Radiology* 1996;198:573–578.
28. Vining DJ, Zagoria RJ, Liu K, Stelts D. CT cystoscopy: an innovation in bladder imaging. *AJR* 1996;166: 409–410.
29. Sommer FG, Olcott EW, Ch'en IY, Beaulieu CF. Volume rendering of CT data: applications to the genitourinary tract. *AJR* 1997;168:1223–1226.

Protocol 1:
BRONCHIAL TREE (Fig. 1)

INDICATION: *Intrabronchial masses, extrinsic compression of bronchi, bronchial strictures*

X-RAY TUBE PARAMETERS: kVp: 120–140
mAs: 220–300

ORAL CONTRAST: None

PHASE OF RESPIRATION: Suspended inspiration after hyperventilation

COLLIMATION: 1–2 mm

PITCH: 1.5–2.0

HELICAL EXPOSURE TIME: 25–40 sec

RECONSTRUCTION INTERVAL: 50% of collimator width (0.5–1 mm)
180-degree linear interpolation

SUPERIOR EXTENT: 2 cm superior to the tracheal carina

INFERIOR EXTENT: 10–12 cm below superior extent

IV CONTRAST: None

COMMENTS:
1. One-mm collimation is preferred, but adequate coverage requires longer (35–40-sec breath-holds) and/or subsecond gantry rotation.
2. Caudal-to-cranial scanning minimizes breathing artifacts near the diaphragm.
3. Reconstruction field of view 18–20 cm, standard kernel.
4. Review for respiratory motion artifacts and rescan if necessary.

SEGMENTATION: None

VISUALIZATION: Curved planar reformations (can be augmented with oblique orthogonal reformations)
External surface displays (central airways only)
  Upper threshold: −700 to −350 HU
Internal surface displays or volume rendering
  Lower threshold/transition zone: −900 HU

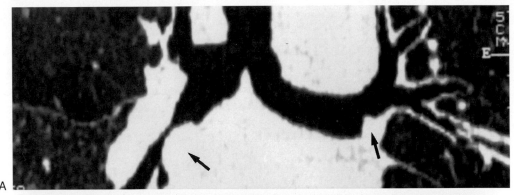

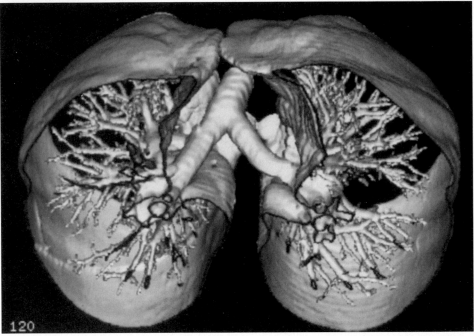

FIG. 1. (**A**) Curved planar reformation in a patient 1 year post heart–lung transplant, demonstrating granulation tissue within the right lower lobe and horizontal portion of the left main stem bronchi (*arrows*). Curved planar reformations facilitate visualization of subtle intraluminal filling defects that may be missed on transverse sections. (Reprinted from Rubin GD. Techniques of reconstruction in spiral CT of the chest. In: M. Rémy-Jardin and J. Rémy, eds., *Spiral CT of the chest*. Berlin: Springer-Verlag, 1996.) (**B**) SR created with an upper threshold of − 150 HU and a lower threshold of − 600 HU clearly demonstrate the distal trachea, mainstem bronchi, and proximal lobar bronchi. The selection of thresholds that render surfaces at the interface between air and soft tissue results in visualization of the central airways within the mediastinum, but within the lung only the vasculature and pleural surface is seen.

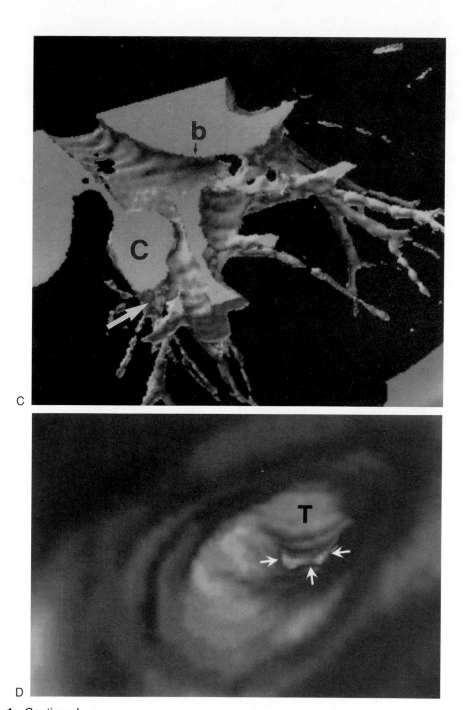

FIG. 1. *Continued.*
(**C**) Sagittal oblique SR with an oblique cut-plane, parallel to the bronchus demonstrates the relationship of a left lower lobe bronchial carcinoid (c) to the left upper lobe bronchus (b) and the superior segmental bronchus of the left lower lobe (arrow). This image facilitated surgical planning, demonstrating that a left lower lobectomy was possible and a total pneumonectomy need not be performed. (Reprinted from Rubin GD. Techniques of reconstruction in spiral CT of the chest. In: M. Rémy-Jardin and J. Rémy, eds., *Spiral CT of the chest.* Berlin: Springer-Verlag, 1996.) (**D**) Perspective volume rendering within the right main stem bronchus looking inferolaterally demonstrates an adenocarcinoma (T), which is markedly narrowing the bronchus intermedius (*arrows*). (Reprinted from Rubin GD. Techniques of reconstruction in spiral CT of the chest. In: M. Rémy-Jardin and J. Rémy, eds., *Spiral CT of the chest.* Berlin: Springer-Verlag, 1996.)

Protocol 2:
LARYNX/CERVICAL TRACHEA (Fig. 2)

INDICATION: *Laryngeal/tracheal masses, tracheal malacia, tracheal strictures*

X-RAY TUBE PARAMETERS: kVp: 120–140
mAs: 220–250

ORAL CONTRAST: None

PHASE OF RESPIRATION: Suspended inspiration after hyperventilation

COLLIMATION: 1–2 mm

PITCH: 1.5–2.0

HELICAL EXPOSURE TIME: 25–40 sec

RECONSTRUCTION INTERVAL: 50% of collimator width (0.5–1 mm)
180-degree linear interpolation

SUPERIOR EXTENT: Base of tongue

INFERIOR EXTENT: Clavicular heads

IV CONTRAST: None

COMMENTS:
1. One-mm collimation is preferred, but adequate coverage requires longer (35–40-sec breath-holds) and/or subsecond gantry rotation.
2. Reconstruction field of view 18–20 cm, standard kernel.
3. Review for motion artifacts and rescan if necessary.

SEGMENTATION: None

VISUALIZATION: Sagittal and coronal oblique reformations
External surface displays
  Upper threshold: −350 HU
Internal surface displays or volume rendering
  Lower threshold/transition zone: −700 to −500 HU

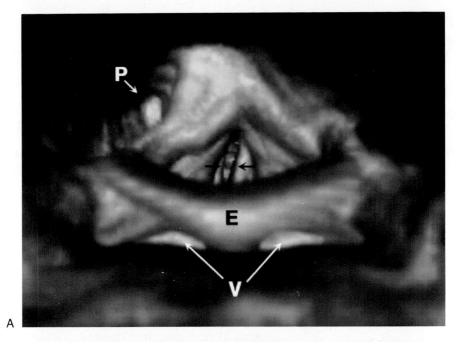

A

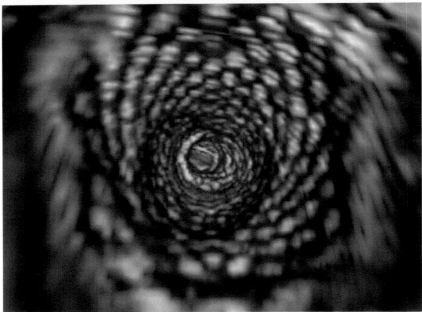

B

FIG. 2. (**A**) Perspective volume rendering of the normal larynx with delineation of the true vocal cords (*black arrows*), epiglottis (E), valleculae (V), and the left pyriform sinus (P). (Reprinted from Rubin GD, Beaulieu CF, Argiro V, et al. Perspective volume rendering of CT and MR images: applications for endoscopic imaging. *Radiology* 1996;199:321–330.) (**B**) Perspective volume rendering within the proximal trachea looking inferiorly through a Wall stent placed to treat a high-grade tracheal stenosis. The tracheal lumen is widely patent. (Reprinted from Rubin GD. Techniques of reconstruction in spiral CT of the chest. In: M. Rémy-Jardin and J. Rémy, eds., *Spiral CT of the chest.* Berlin: Springer-Verlag, 1996.)

Protocol 3:
COLON (Fig. 3)

INDICATION:	*Colonic polyps, neoplasia, and strictures*
X-RAY TUBE PARAMETERS:	kVp: 120–140 mAs: 250–320
BOWEL PREPARATION:	One gallon of Golytely (Braintree, Braintree, MA) or similar preparation drunk day before the exam over a 4-hr period or 1.5 oz evening before and 1.5 oz Fleet Phosphosoda 3 hr prior to exam. Both protocols: clear liquids day of exam and NPO 3 hr prior to exam
ORAL CONTRAST:	None
RECTAL CONTRAST:	Air insufflation via 12–16 Fr. rubber tube
PHASE OF RESPIRATION:	Suspended inspiration after hyperventilation as long as possible, then quiet ventilation
COLLIMATION:	3 mm
PITCH:	2.0, 180-degree linear interpolation
HELICAL EXPOSURE TIME:	50–60 sec
RECONSTRUCTION INTERVAL:	50% of collimator width (1.5 mm)
SUPERIOR EXTENT:	1 cm above upper extent of colon on scout
INFERIOR EXTENT:	Anus
IV CONTRAST:	None
COMMENTS:	1. Reconstruction field of view to include colon, standard kernel. 2. Review for incomplete distention, particularly in the sigmoid colon, and consider rescanning of undistended segments or segments with retained fluid: prone to cover sigmoid colon and cecum from iliac crest to rectum.
SEGMENTATION:	None
VISUALIZATION:	Curved planar reformations (can be augmented with oblique orthonormal to color reformations) External surface displays (central airways only) Upper threshold: −700 to −350 HU Internal surface displays or volume rendering Lower threshold/transition zone: −850–900 HU

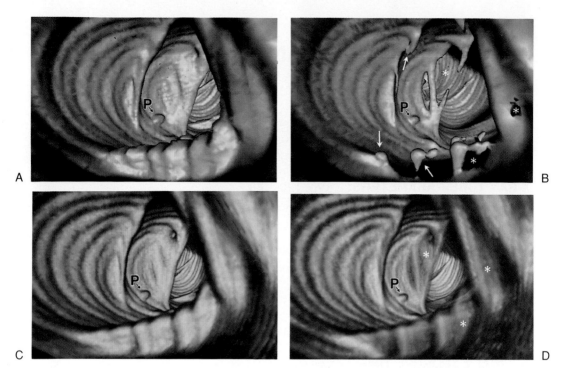

FIG. 3. (**A**) Perspective shaded-surface display of colonic helical CT with threshold of −980 HU, which is optimal for displaying the interior of the colon, and (**B**) threshold of −930 HU, which is too high. Portions of the colonic wall are not rendered and present as holes (*) or intraluminal juxtamural structures (*arrows*) that could be misinterpreted as polyps. A 5-mm polyp is visible in all views (P). (**C**) Perspective volume rendering with an opacity curve that renders all voxels above −980 as 80% to 100% opaque is free from both artifactual wall discontinuities and juxtamural structures. (**D**) Perspective volume rendering with a different-opacity curve that renders the lower densities more transparently, creates a wispy appearance of the thinner structures (*). Frank discontinuities as seen with surface displays are not created. The presence of semitransparent cues on volume-rendered images (**C,D**) results in easier detection of errors than on surface displays (**A,B**). Once detected, the opacity curve can be adjusted and the image rerendered in 10−20 sec. (Reprinted from Rubin GD, Beaulieu CF, Argiro V, et al. Perspective volume rendering of CT and MR images: applications for endoscopic imaging. *Radiology* 1996;199:321−330.)

Protocol 4:
INTRACRANIAL CT ANGIOGRAPHY
(Fig. 4)

INDICATION:	*Aneurysms or arterial occlusive disease from atherosclerosis, atheroembolization, or dissection*
X-RAY TUBE PARAMETERS:	kVp: 120–140 mAs: 250–300
ORAL CONTRAST:	None
PHASE OF RESPIRATION:	Quiet ventilation
COLLIMATION:	1 mm
PITCH:	2.0, 180-degree linear interpolation
HELICAL EXPOSURE TIME:	25–40 sec
RECONSTRUCTION INTERVAL:	50% of collimator width (0.5 mm)
SUPERIOR EXTENT:	6–8 cm above foramen magnum
INFERIOR EXTENT:	Foramen magnum

IV CONTRAST:

Concentration:	LOCM 300–320 mg iodine/mL
Rate:	3–4 mL/sec
Scan Delay:	Timed in internal carotid arteries
Total Volume:	120–160 mL

COMMENTS:

1. Scan caudal to cranial to avoid cavernous carotid obscuration from filling of the cavernous sinus.
2. Angle gantry (10–20 degrees) to avoid superimposition of artifacts from dental fillings onto pertinent vasculature.
3. Reconstruction field of view 10–15 cm, standard kernel.

SEGMENTATION: Usually unnecessary for STS-MIP, superior to inferior orthographic SR/VR, and all perspective renderings.

ROI or region growing can be used to remove anterior, posterior, and lateral margins of the skull.

If base of skull subtraction is necessary, then region growing can identify and subtract skull; however, this can be difficult and may require additional localized ROI editing to disconnect skull base from blood vessels in some regions.

VISUALIZATION: STS-MIP transverse, coronal

Orthographic and external perspective surface or volume renderings (external perspective rendering eliminates necessity of segmentation)

Upper threshold: 150–300 HU

Internal surface or volume rendering

Lower threshold: 150–250 HU

FIG. 4. (**A**) Sagittal slab-MIP throughout the anterior circle of Willis, demonstrating a large aneurysm (*arrow*) of the anterior communicating artery. (**B**) Perspective SR from within the posterior cranium shows the middle cerebral arteries (*short arrows*), the anterior cerebral arteries (*long arrows*), and active extravasation of contrast material (*long curved arrow*) from a teat (*short curved arrow*) at the apex of the aneurysm. (Reprinted with permission from Gosselin MV, Vieco PT. Active hemorrhage of intracranial aneurysms: diagnosis by CT angiography. *JCAT* 1997;21:22–24.)

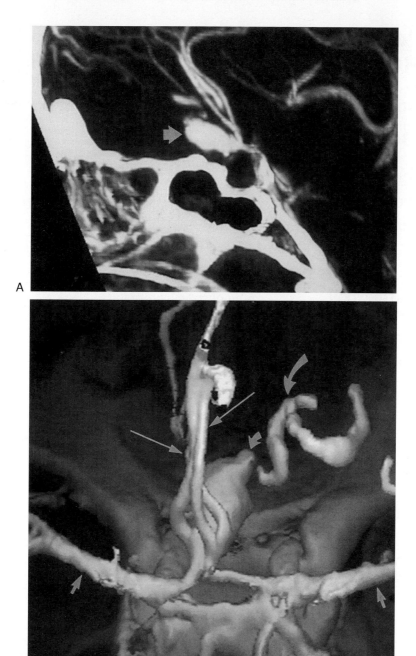

Protocol 5:
CAROTID ARTERY BIFURCATION (Fig. 5)

INDICATION:	*Atherosclerotic occlusive disease or dissection*
X-RAY TUBE PARAMETERS:	kVp: 120–140 mAs: 220–300
ORAL CONTRAST:	None
PHASE OF RESPIRATION:	Suspended inspiration after hyperventilation
COLLIMATION:	2–3 mm
PITCH:	1.5–2.0, 180-degree linear interpolation
HELICAL EXPOSURE TIME:	25–40 sec
RECONSTRUCTION INTERVAL:	50% of collimator width (1–1.5 mm)
SUPERIOR EXTENT:	Base of skull
INFERIOR EXTENT:	Base of neck

IV CONTRAST:

Concentration:	LOCM 300–320 mg iodine/mL
Rate:	3–4 mL/sec
Scan Delay:	Timed in internal carotid arteries
Total Volume:	120–160 mL

COMMENTS:
1. Reconstruction field of view 15 cm, standard kernel.
2. Caudal-to-cranial scan direction

SEGMENTATION:
None for CPR or STS-MIP
Bone removal by region growing or ROI editing. For removal of opacified jugular vein (orthographic surface and volume renderings) additional detailed ROI editing to disconnect carotid arteries from jugular veins prior to removal by region growing.

VISUALIZATION:
Curved planar reformations, STS-MIP (oblique)
External surface displays (limited utility, especially when calcium is present)
Upper threshold: 100–200 HU

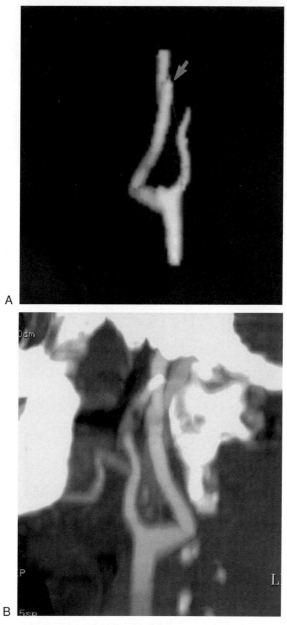

FIG. 5. (**A**) SR of the left common carotid bifurcation demonstrates a tortuous and kinked proximal internal carotid artery with a small pseudoaneurysm (*arrow*) of the internal carotid artery status post repair of carotid dissection. The carotid arteries were isolated by a combination of region growing and three-dimensional ROI editing. (**B**) Curved planar reformation demonstrates the same lesions but did not require preliminary editing.

Protocol 6:
CAROTID ARTERY ORIGIN TO SKULL BASE AND VERTEBRAL ARTERIES
(Fig. 6)

INDICATION:	*Detection of tandem atherosclerotic occlusive disease or extensive dissection*
X-RAY TUBE PARAMETERS:	kVp: 120–140 mAs: 220–300
ORAL CONTRAST:	None
PHASE OF RESPIRATION:	Suspended inspiration after hyperventilation
COLLIMATION:	3 mm
PITCH:	2.0, 180-degree linear interpolation
HELICAL EXPOSURE TIME:	40 sec
RECONSTRUCTION INTERVAL:	50% of collimator width (1.5 mm)
SUPERIOR EXTENT:	Base of skull
INFERIOR EXTENT:	Mid-aortic arch

IV CONTRAST:

Concentration:	LOCM 300–320 mg iodine/mL
Rate:	3–4 mL/sec
Scan Delay:	Timed in aortic arch
Total Volume:	120–160 mL

COMMENTS:

1. Venous access via right upper extremity.
2. Reconstruction field of view 24 cm, standard kernel.

SEGMENTATION:

None for CPR or STS-MIP
Bone removal by region growing or ROI editing. For removal of opacified jugular vein (orthographic surface and volume renderings) additional detailed ROI editing to disconnect carotid arteries from jugular veins prior to removal by region growing.

VISUALIZATION:
Curved planar reformations (carotids and
vertebral arteries)
Oblique STS-MIP (carotids only)
External surface displays (limited utility,
especially when calcium is present)
Upper threshold: 100–200 HU

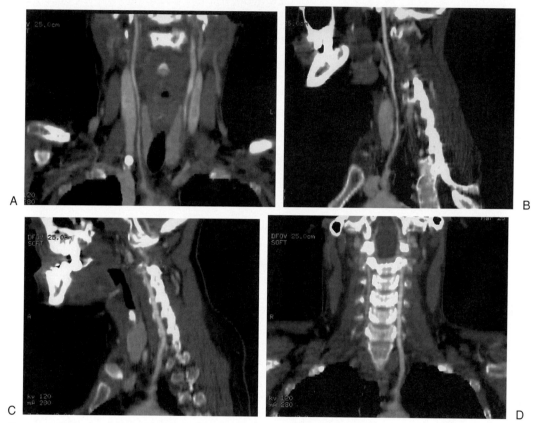

FIG. 6. Curved planar reformations of the right common and internal carotid arteries (**A,B**) from the origin of the common carotid artery to the skull base in a patient with diffuse carotid artery stenosis from Takayasu arteritis. Mural thickening is evident in the common carotid artery on both views. When using curved planar reformations, it is important to create two orthogonal views, in this case curved coronal and curved sagittal, to allow visualization of eccentric lesions. Curved sagittal (**C**) and curved coronal (**D**) reformations through the left vertebral artery demonstrate this large vessel through its entire course, including the cervical portion through the foramen transversaria of C1–C6. Other external displays of this vessel would require highly labor-intensive and artifact-producing editing of the vertebrae from the artery.

Protocol 7:
THORACIC AORTA (Fig. 7)

INDICATION:	*Aneurysm, dissection, mural hematoma/ ulceration, trauma, coarctation, anomalies*
X-RAY TUBE PARAMETERS:	kVp: 120–140 mAs: 250–300
ORAL CONTRAST:	None
PHASE OF RESPIRATION:	Suspended inspiration after hyperventilation
COLLIMATION:	3 mm
PITCH:	1.5–2.0, 180-degree linear interpolation
HELICAL EXPOSURE TIME:	30–40 sec
RECONSTRUCTION INTERVAL:	50% of collimator width (1.5 mm)
SUPERIOR EXTENT:	4 cm above top of aortic arch
INFERIOR EXTENT:	As low as necessary to image lesion. If dissection extends into abdomen, then a second acquisition is typically required.

IV CONTRAST:

Concentration:	LOCM 300–320 mg iodine/mL
Rate:	3–4 mL/sec
Scan Delay:	Timed in aortic arch (time both true and false lumen in presence of dissection and select intermediate delay time)
Total Volume:	120–160 mL

COMMENTS:	1. Venous access via right upper extremity 2. Reconstruction field of view 24 cm, standard kernel.
SEGMENTATION:	None for CPR Bone removal by ROI editing for SR.
VISUALIZATION:	Curved planar reformations External surface or volume renderings (MIP rarely useful for the thoracic aorta) Upper threshold/transition zone: 150–300 HU

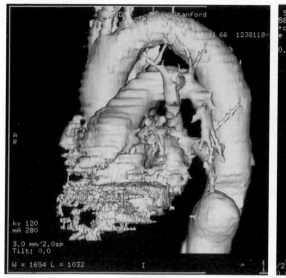
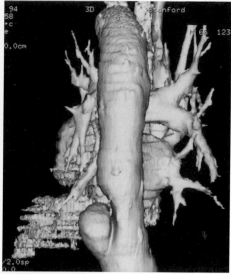
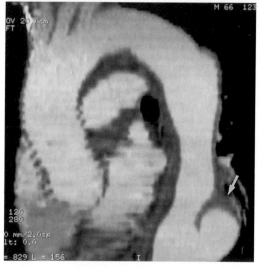

FIG. 7. (**A**) Left lateral and (**B**) posterior shaded-surface displays of a spiral CT angiogram—obtained with 3-mm collimation, 2.0 pitch, and 2-mm reconstruction interval—demonstrate a penetrating ulcer on the left lateral wall of the descending thoracic aorta. Mass effect, suggestive of thrombus, is observed on the aorta just proximal to the ulceration. (**C**) Curved planar reformation enables delineation of both the patent portion of the intramural ulceration and the superior thrombosed portion (*arrow*); however, considerable distortion results from curved drawing, which erroneously gives the impression that the ulceration is on the posterior wall. Curved planar reformations must always be reviewed in association with transverse sections, maximum-intensity projections, or shaded-surface displays to clarify where regions of anatomic distortion might exist. (Reprinted from Rubin GD. Techniques of reconstruction in spiral CT of the chest. In: M. Rémy-Jardin and J. Rémy, eds., *Spiral CT of the chest.* Berlin: Springer-Verlag, 1996.)

Protocol 8:
ABDOMINAL AORTA AND ILIAC ARTERIES (Fig. 8)

INDICATION:	*Aneurysm, atherosclerotic occlusive disease, and dissection*
X-RAY TUBE PARAMETERS:	kVp: 120–140 mAs: 220–300
ORAL CONTRAST:	None
PHASE OF RESPIRATION:	Suspended inspiration after hyperventilation for first 30–40 sec, then quiet ventilation
COLLIMATION:	1-sec gantry rotation: 3 mm from supraceliac through renal arteries, then 5 mm to inguinal ligament 0.75-sec gantry rotation: 3 mm throughout
PITCH:	2.0, 180-degree linear interpolation
HELICAL EXPOSURE TIME:	45–55 sec
RECONSTRUCTION INTERVAL:	50% of collimator width (1.5–2.5 mm)
SUPERIOR EXTENT:	1–2 cm above celiac origin
INFERIOR EXTENT:	Lesser trochanter of femur

IV CONTRAST:

Concentration:	LOCM 300–320 mg iodine/mL
Rate:	4 mL/sec
Scan Delay:	Timed in supraceliac aorta
Total Volume:	160–190 mL

COMMENTS:

1. Suspended inspiration to continue through scan delay, while collination changes from 3 to 5 mm.
2. Reconstruction field of view = total table travel distance, standard kernel of entire data set
3. Reconstruction field of view 20 cm, standard kernel through renal arteries.

SEGMENTATION:

None for CPR
Bone removal:
1. Highest threshold to isolate blood vessels and bones without losing important aortic branches

2. ROI editing to disconnect arteries and bones (typically superior gluteal arteries exiting pelvis and regions of lumbar osteophytes)
3. Region growing remove blood vessels
4. Dilation 3–5 pixels
5. Subtraction (Boolean operation) of resultant data set from original data

Note: If technique described is unavailable, then more time-consuming ROI editing is necessary.

Additional limited ROI or region growing removal of venous structures and celiac/mesenteric arterial branches may occasionally be necessary.

VISUALIZATION:

Curved planar reformations
External surface or volume renderings
Upper threshold/transition zone: 150–300 HU
MIP (visualization of calcified plaque an external wall of aneurysm and other arteries)

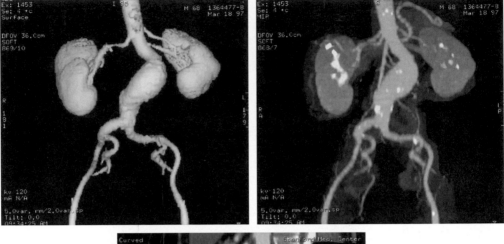

A   B

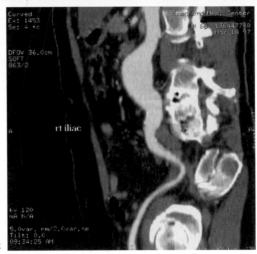

C

FIG. 8. (A) SR demonstrates an infrarenal AAA. **(B)** MIP allows easier differentiation of the less opacified left renal vein from the left renal artery, and calcified atheroma on the wall of the aorta and iliac arteries is visible. Cues to depth relationships in the tortuous right external iliac artery are not evident. **(C)** Curved planar reformation displays abdominal aorta and right iliac without preliminary editing.

Protocol 9:
COMBINED THORACIC AND ABDOMINAL AORTA

INDICATION: *Aneurysm or dissection*

X-RAY TUBE PARAMETERS: kVp: 120–140
mAs: 250–300

ORAL CONTRAST: None

PHASE OF RESPIRATION: Suspended inspiration after hyperventilation for first 30–40 sec, then quiet ventilation in abdomen. Suspended inspiration after hyperventilation in chest

COLLIMATION: Abdomen: 3 mm
Chest: 3–5 mm in chest, depending on contrast usage limitations

PITCH: 2.0

HELICAL EXPOSURE TIME: Abdomen: 30–40 sec
Chest: 20–30 sec

RECONSTRUCTION INTERVAL: 50% of collimator width (1.5–2.5 mm)

SUPERIOR EXTENT: 2 cm above aortic arch

INFERIOR EXTENT: Below aortic bifurcation, as necessary

IV CONTRAST:

Concentration:	LOCM 300–320 mg iodine/mL
Rate:	4 mL/sec
Scan Delay:	Timed in supraceliac aorta
Total Volume:	250–300 mL

COMMENTS:
1. The abdomen is scanned first, prior to arterial obscuration, by venous, parenchymal, or ureteral opacification. The power injector typically requires reloading with 50–100 mL of contrast between scans.
2. Contrast utilization must be weighed against improved spatial resolution and/or anatomic coverage.

SEGMENTATION: Chest: same as for thoracic aorta
Abdomen: same as for abdominal aorta

VISUALIZATION: Chest: same as for thoracic aorta
Abdomen: same as for abdominal aorta

Protocol 10:
RENAL ARTERIES (Fig. 9)

INDICATION: *Atherosclerotic occlusive disease, assessment of potential living renal donors*

X-RAY TUBE PARAMETERS: kVp: 120–140
mAs: 250–300

ORAL CONTRAST: None

PHASE OF RESPIRATION: Suspended inspiration after hyperventilation

COLLIMATION: 2–3 mm

PITCH: 1.5–2.0, 180-degree linear interpolation

HELICAL EXPOSURE TIME: 30–40 sec

RECONSTRUCTION INTERVAL: 50% of collimator width (1–1.5 mm)

SUPERIOR EXTENT: Superior aspect of kidneys or superior mesenteric artery, whichever is more cephalad.

INFERIOR EXTENT: Inferior aspect of kidneys or to common iliac bifurcation, whichever is more caudal.

IV CONTRAST:

Concentration:	LOCM 300–320 mg iodine/mL
Rate:	4–5 mL/sec
Scan Delay:	Timed in abdominal aorta
Total Volume:	120–160 mL

COMMENTS:
1. Reconstruction field of view 18–24 cm, standard kernel.
2. Delayed scout with 80 kV obtained 5 min after injection in potential renal donors. Repeat once if ureteral opacification is inadequate.

SEGMENTATION: None for CPR and STS-MIP
Bone removal by ROI editing for SR/VR and MIP

VISUALIZATION: Curved planar reformations (best for stenosis
                          associated with calcification; must have curved
                          coronal and curved transverse reformations to
                          assess eccentric plaque)
                          STS-MIP
                          SR/VR (renal donors only)
                             Upper threshold: 150–300 HU
                          MIP (as needed)

FIG. 9. (A) SR of the aorta and renal arteries. The gray scale encodes depth. All visualized pixels were above an arbitrary threshold value. Calcification at the origins of the renal arteries is seen as a contour abnormality (*arrows*). **(B)** MIP in the same patient. Gray scale encodes CT number. There is no depth encoding. Calcium is brighter because of its greater x-ray attenuation. Left renal arterial calcium appears to completely occlude the lumen in this view. **(C)** One-pixel-thick curved planar reformation demonstrates eccentric mural calcification of the proximal renal arteries bilaterally. The left renal arterial origin calcification is shown to be nonocclusive (*straight arrow*). **(D)** Curved planar reformation, reconstructed from a slightly different curve, completely eliminates the mural calcification from the arteries, attesting to the eccentricity of the calcified plaque and the absence of significant renal artery stenosis. The lumenal narrowing in the right renal artery (*curved arrow*) is spurious because of inaccurate curve drawing. (Reprinted from Rubin GD, Dake MD, Semba CS. Current status of 3-D spiral CT for imaging the vasculature. *Radiol Clin North Am* 1995;33:51–70.)

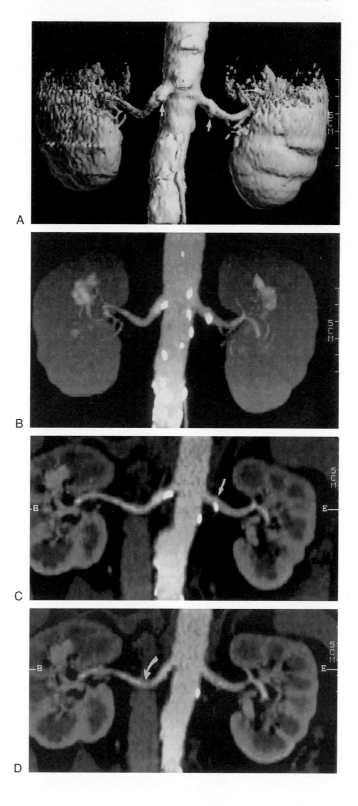

Protocol 11:
SPLANCHNIC ARTERIES AND VEINS
(Fig. 10)

INDICATION: *Chronic mesenteric ischemia, aneurysms, invasion by neoplasm, preoperative detection of anomalous hepatic arterial supply*

X-RAY TUBE PARAMETERS: kVp: 120–140
mAs: 250–300

ORAL CONTRAST: None

PHASE OF RESPIRATION: Suspended inspiration after hyperventilation

COLLIMATION: 2–3 mm

PITCH: 1.5–2.0, 180-degree linear interpolation

HELICAL EXPOSURE TIME: 30 sec

RECONSTRUCTION INTERVAL: 50% of collimator width (1–1.5 mm)

SUPERIOR EXTENT: 2 cm above celiac origin

INFERIOR EXTENT: Inferior aspect of pancreas

IV CONTRAST:

Concentration:	LOCM 300–320 mg iodine/mL
Rate:	4–5 mL/sec
Scan Delay:	Timed in abdominal aorta
Total Volume:	120–160 mL

COMMENTS:
1. Reconstruction field of view 18 cm, standard kernel.
2. A second scan obtained with similar parameters 10 sec after the arterial acquisition may be useful in the setting of neoplasm to display portal, splenic, and superior mesenteric venous involvement and venous collateral pathways.

SEGMENTATION: None for CPR and STS-MIP
Bone removal by ROI or region growing for SR/VR

VISUALIZATION: Curved planar reformations (best for stenosis
                           associated with calcification; must have curved
                           coronal and curved transverse reformations to
                           assess eccentric plaque)
                        Oblique, sagittal, and/or coronal MPR for
                           depicting relationship between neoplasia
                           and arteries
                        STS-MIP
                        SR/VR (preop planning):
                           Upper threshold/transition zone: 150–300 HU

FIG. 10. (**A**) SR of normal splanchnic circulation shows aorta (A), splenic artery (s), hepatic artery (*open arrow*), splenic vein (sv), and portal vein (p). Renal arteries with stenosis of left renal artery origin (*curved arrows*) and renal veins (*straight arrows*) entering inferior vena cava (i) are also demonstrated. (Reprinted from Rubin GD, Walker PJ, Dake MD, et al. 3-D spiral CT angiography: an alternate imaging modality for the abdominal aorta and its branches. *J Vasc Surg* 1993;18:656–666). (**B**) Frontal MIP-CTA demonstrates distal superior mesenteric venous occlusion (*curved arrow*) with extensive collaterals supplying the pancreatico-duodenal branch that reconstitutes the extrahepatic portal vein (p). An abnormally enlarged coronary vein (*long arrow*) drains extensive gastric varices (*short arrows*). Complete occlusion of the splenic vein is additionally established. (Reprinted from Rubin GD, Jeffrey RB. 3-D spiral CT angiography of the abdomen and thorax. In: Fishman EK, Jeffrey RB, eds. *Spiral CT principles, techniques and clinical application.* New York: Raven Press 1994;183–196).

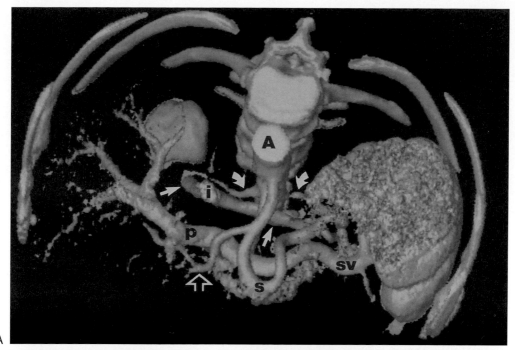

A

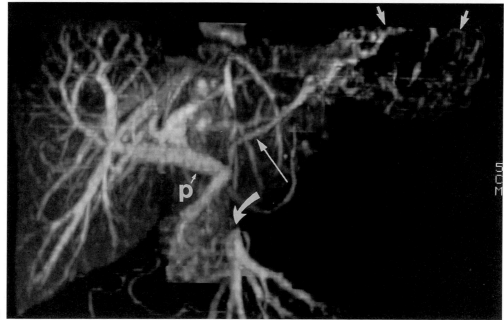

B

Protocol 12:
EXTREMITY CTA

INDICATION: *Trauma*

X-RAY TUBE PARAMETERS: kVp: 120–140
mAs: 220–250

ORAL CONTRAST: None

PHASE OF RESPIRATION: Breathing

COLLIMATION: 1–3 mm

PITCH: 1.5–2.0, 180-degree linear interpolation

HELICAL EXPOSURE TIME: 30–40 sec

RECONSTRUCTION INTERVAL: 50% of collimator width (0.5–1.5 mm)

SUPERIOR EXTENT: 2–4 cm above suspected lesion

INFERIOR EXTENT: 2–4 cm below suspected lesion

IV CONTRAST:

Concentration:	LOCM 300–320 mg iodine/mL
Rate:	3–4 mL/sec
Scan Delay:	Timed in artery of interest
Total Volume:	120–160 mL

COMMENTS:
1. Venous access not into extremity of interest.
2. Reconstruction field of view 15–24 cm, standard kernel.

SEGMENTATION: None for CPR or SSD/VR (it is frequently useful to display bony landmarks adjacent to vascular lesions for localization
Bone removal by ROI or region growing as needed

VISUALIZATION: Curved planar reformations
SSD/VR
Upper threshold/transition zone: 150–300 HU

Subject Index

Subject Index